NATURAL & ARTIFICIAL PARALLEL COMPUTATION

Proceedings of the Fifth
NEC Research Symposium

Proceedings of the NEC Research Symposia

Gear, C. W., *Computation & Cognition: Proceedings of the First NEC Research Symposium*

Ishiguro, T., *Algorithms & Architectures: Proceedings of the Second NEC Research Symposium*

Baum, Eric B., *Computational Learning & Cognition: Proceedings of the Third NEC Research Symposium*

Ishiguro, T., *Cognitive Processing for Vision & Voice: Proceedings of the Fourth NEC Research Symposium*

Waltz, David L., *Natural & Artificial Parallel Computation: Proceedings of the Fifth NEC Research Symposium*

NATURAL *&* ARTIFICIAL
PARALLEL COMPUTATION

Proceedings of the Fifth
NEC Research Symposium

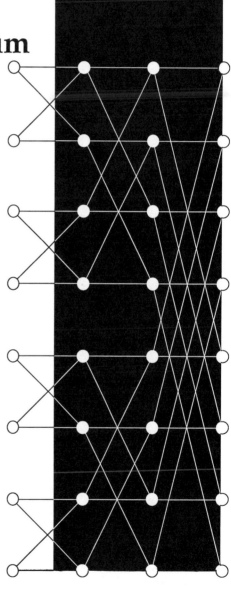

Society for Industrial and Applied Mathematics
Philadelphia

Edited by
David L. Waltz

Library of Congress Cataloging-in-Publication Data

NEC Research Symposium (5th : 1994 : Princeton, N.J.)
     Natural & artificial parallel computation : proceedings of the
fifth NEC Research Symposium / edited by David L. Waltz.
     p.   cm .
     Includes bibliographical references and index.
     ISBN 0-89871-357-9
     1. Parallel processing (Electronic computers)--Congresses.
I. Waltz, David L.
QA76.58.N43 1996
004'.35—dc20   95-48918

Preface

The Fifth NEC Research Symposium coincided with the fifth anniversary of the NEC Research Institute. For this occasion, we picked a topic — Natural and Artificial Parallel Computation — that covers many of the central issues that NECI was chartered to investigate and advance.

It would have been difficult to foresee at the time of NECI's founding just how rapidly computer science and computational neuroscience would converge. Neuroscience seems to be advancing at a breakneck pace, comparable to that of the computing industry. Neuroscience progress has been spurred in part by advances in instrumentation — MRI and CAT scanners of ever-greater resolution and single-cell and multiple-cell recording equipment, in particular. Neuroscience is also being driven by rapid increases in computing power, which have brought ever-larger problems within the range of solution. For example, accurate simulation of individual neurons and neural assemblies is now possible. But in addition, the rapid growth of neuroscience has caused scientists to become aware of the need for new theoretical frameworks that can encompass both natural and artificial computation. We are just beginning to see the influence our increased understanding in neuroscience has on computer science; an early example of this influence is massively parallel processing (MPP), a topic of great interest in the computing industry. The central question of MPP, similar to the central question of neuroscience, is this: how can a very large number of relatively slow components work together to provide very rapid solutions to large problems? Finally, computer scientists increasingly draw inspiration from the evolution of populations of entities.

This volume contains papers by world experts on topics that span the range of these questions and issues. It begins with processing in biological organisms, moves through interactions between biology and computer science, and ends with massively parallel computing. Catherine Carr's paper discusses the time-based processing used by electric fish and barn owls to navigate and locate prey. Rob de Ruyter and his coauthors discuss research on the visual processing employed by flies to control navigation. Larry Abbott and his coauthors describe detailed simulation of a neuron — a simulation accurate enough that a computer running the simulation can be inserted into a neural assembly in place of a neuron and the overall function of the assembly will be retained. Tom Ray describes Tierra, his evolutionary digital universe, where parasites and hyperparasites evolve, shedding light on hypothesized processes of evolution such as punctuated equilibrium. Shigeru Tanaka describes the self-organization of cells in the primary visual cortex and the light that this sheds on information representation in the brain. Les Valiant presents a framework for modeling very large networks of "neuroids," i.e., abstract neurons. His model can scale to the size of real brains but is at the same time mathematically tractable, so that it is possible to prove results about the complexity of various operations, e.g., classical conditioning. Akihiko Konagaya describes his work in using AI learning algorithms — based on the MDL (minimum description length) principle and genetic algorithms — to solve important problems in locating motifs in genetic sequences. Bill Dally discusses the many factors — especially bandwidth, node granularity, and communication mechanisms — and engineering trade-offs among them that must be addressed when building massively parallel machines. Finally Shuichi Sakai describes design issues for the massively parallel machine being built by the Japanese Real World Computing Project.

I would like to thank the many people who helped make the symposium on which this book is based a success. Although it is impossible to mention everyone, I would especially like to acknowledge all of the speakers/authors; Nobuhiko Koike of NEC, who selected and arranged for the participation of the authors from Japan; Steve Oppen, who ably chaired the Local Arrangements Committee and personally handled many of the arrangements; and Irene Parker, my secretary and member of the Local Arrangements Committee, who kept track of everything for me, thereby averting any number of potential disasters.

David L. Waltz
Princeton, 1995

Contents

Time Coding in the CNS 1
Catherine E. Carr

Adaptive Movement Computation by the Blowfly Visual System 21
R. R. de Ruyter van Steveninck, W. Bialek, M. Potters, R. H. Carlson,
and G. D. Lewen

Activity-Dependent Conductances in Model and Biological Neurons 43
L.F. Abbott, G. Turrigiano, G. LeMasson, and E. Marder

Evolution of Parallel Processes in Organic and Digital Media 69
Thomas S. Ray

Information Representation and Self-Organization of the
Primary Visual Cortex 93
Shigeru Tanaka

A Neuroidal Model for Cognition 127
Leslie G. Valiant

Knowledge Discovery in Genetic Sequences 141
Akihiko Konagaya

Bandwidth, Granularity, and Mechanisms: Key Issues in the
Design of Parallel Computers 163
William J. Dally

RWC Massively Parallel Computer Project: RWC Architecture 183
Shuichi Sakai

Index 197

Chapter 1
Time Coding in the CNS[*]

Catherine E. Carr[‡]

Abstract

Studies of time coding in the central nervous system have revealed circuits specialized for the encoding and processing of microsecond time differences in two specialists, weakly electric fish and barn owls. These animals can detect microsecond time differences, and analysis of how they process temporal information has uncovered many common principles. Despite their different neural substrates, time coding systems share similar features and implement similar algorithms for the encoding of temporal information. Timing information is generally coded by phase-locked action potentials, and processed in a dedicated pathway **in parallel** with other stimulus variables. The elements of time-coding circuits have morphological and physiological features suited to their function. These circuits also show increasing specializations for the extraction of relevant temporal features needed to measure temporal cues such as time differences. Information from the parallel channels is later recombined in higher centers for the computation of relevant stimulus features.

1   Introduction

Information is processed in parallel in all sensory systems. In most senses, a dichotomy exists between coding for the timing or phase of the signal and coding for its amplitude. In the visual system, for example, the separation of information into two channels which differ in their spatial and temporal acuity begins in the retina [22]. The parallel processing of temporal and amplitude information is a defining feature of both the electric sense and the auditory system, and is described in this review. In electric fish, the dichotomy between phase and amplitude coding begins at the receptor level, while in the auditory system the separation into phase and amplitude coding is

---

[*]This work was supported by an Alfred P. Sloan Fellowship and by NIH grant DCD000436. This chapter builds on an earlier review in the Annual Review of Neurocience (1993).

[‡] Department of Zoology, University of Maryland, College Park, MD 20742-4415, USA.

derived within the central nervous system. Despite these different neural substrates, the CNS time channels share numerous morphological and physiological adaptations to improve the time-coding of signal. Accurate coding of temporal information is widespread in the central nervous system, and many theories of sensory biology depend upon the detection of signals that are correlated in time. The review describes the major features of time coding systems by concentrating on specialists such as weakly electric fish, barn owls and echolocating bats, because of their well developed abilities to detect time differences.

Analysis of how animals process temporal information has uncovered many common principles. In time coding systems, the timing of the stimulus is coded by phase-locked action potentials, timing information is processed in a dedicated pathway in parallel with other stimulus variables, and the time coding cells have morphological and physiological features suited to their function. Furthermore, time coding circuits show increasing specializations for the extraction of relevant temporal features needed to measure time differences. The circuits that measure time differences in different animals also employ similar algorithms. All circuits that detect time differences depend on some form of delay lines and coincidence detectors, where the coincidence detectors are neurons that respond maximally when they receive simultaneous inputs. This can occur when the time difference is compensated for by delay of the earlier of the two inputs. The coincidence detector circuits use temporal information to compute the new variable of time difference.

2   Behavior and detection of temporal information

When sound comes from one side of the body, it reaches one ear before the other. The brain detects these interaural time differences and translates them into sound location. Various animals show great sensitivity to these small time differences. Nocturnal predators such as owls, bats, and many other mammals are able to detect time differences on the order of 0.5 μsec [11,23,27]. Similar sensitivity to small time differences include the discrimination of phase differences between signals on different parts of the body surface in electric fish [3,33]. The behavioral studies outlined below delineate each animal's ability to detect time differences.

2.1   The Electrosensory System

Weakly electric fish generate an electric field around their body by discharging an electric organ. The field is detected by electroreceptors scattered over the body surface. The electric sense is used for location of objects and for communication with conspecifics. The electric fish, *Eigenmannia*, produces a quasisinusoidal electric organ discharge in the range of 400 - 600 Hz. When these fish encounter neighbours with similar electric organ discharge frequencies, the electric signals add in the water and produce a beating signal which interferes each animal's ability to electrolocate because the small disturbances caused by the presence of a prey item are masked by the large changes in amplitude and phase caused by the interfering signals. When electric fish with similar electric organ discharge frequencies meet, each fish shifts the frequency of its electric organ discharge so as to increase the frequency difference between them [2]. In this jamming avoidance response, the fish determines whether its neighbour has a higher or lower frequency than its own by evaluating the fluctuations in amplitude and phase of the beating signal on different parts of its body surface [13]. Since this behavior requires detection of phase differences, it is an assay for the minimum phase difference that can be perceived by the fish [3,33].

The jamming avoidance response was used to demonstrate that electric fish detect phase differences in the microsecond range [3]. Fish were presented with weaker and weaker jamming stimuli that produced small phase differences between different parts of the body surface (Fig. 1). Jamming avoidance responses to these weak jamming stimuli showed that the fish detect phase differences of about 0.5µs between different parts of the body surface.

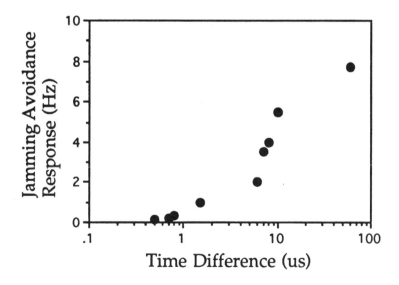

Fig. 1. *Jamming Avoidance Response showing detection of small (05 us) phase differences between different parts of the body surface [from 3].*

2.2   The Auditory System

Barn owl's are able to use auditory cues alone to catch mice in total darkness [20,31]. Sounds from one side of the body reaches one ear before the other, and these interaural time differences are translated into location in azimuth. The owl does not use the time of arrival or onset of the sound, but uses the phase differences between the two ears [27]. Interaural time differences are then derived from the interaural phase differences present in the auditory stimulus.

Interaural phase differences are generally the salient cue for localization of low frequency sounds [8,11]. Barn owls have larger heads and thus larger interaural time differences than many birds of similar size and weight. Their large head size may permit a greater resolution of binaural time differences. Sound localization ability is not always well correlated with head size. It is highly correlated with directing the attention of the other senses to the sound source. Animals with narrow fields of best visual acuity require accurate sound localization to direct their gaze [11].

3   Encoding of temporal information

The discrimination of small time differences described in the previous section requires accurate transduction and processing of the original stimulus. Time coding arises in the periphery, and timing information is preserved and improved in the CNS. In addition to precise neural coding, behavioral hyperacuity is assumed to involve averaging in large neural assembles. Both strategies may be found in these time coding systems.

3.1   The Electrosensory System

The electric sense has a comparatively simple organization, with about 15,000 electroreceptors distributed on the fish's body surface. There are two types of electroreceptors, ampullary and tuberous [45]. Ampullary electroreceptors respond to low-frequency AC fields, such as the bioelectric fields produced by prey species, other fish, plants etc. They also respond to the low frequency EOD modulations used in electric fish courtship, and to some fields of inanimate origin.

Tuberous electroreceptors are specialized for the detection of the EOD and are tuned to the fundamental frequency of the EOD. They are more numerous than ampullary receptors, and their distribution over the body surface provides a somatotopically organized view of the electrosensory world that may be best compared with that presented to the visual system by an extended retina without a lens. The high density of electroreceptors enables the system to provide an electric image of the fish's immediate surroundings for electrolocation. Each receptor unit is innervated by a single primary afferent which has its cell body in the ganglion of the anterior lateral line nerve. There are two types of tuberous unit; one encodes modulations in signal *amplitude*, and the other encodes the signal *phase* or timing of every cycle of the EOD [37,45]. Nerve fibers that innervate the phase-coding type of electroreceptors fire one spike on each cycle of the stimulus, phase-locked with little jitter to the zero-crossing of the stimulus.

The segregation of phase and amplitude receptors in the skin is reinforced by the connections formed by their afferents in the medulla. Phase and amplitude coding afferents terminate on different cell types in different laminae of the lateral line lobe, although they remain in somatotopic register. The separation of phase and amplitude information into two parallel channels is a common feature of all time coding systems. In electric fish, the two channels have distinct morphology as well as separate connections. Phase-coding terminals are specialized for maintenance of phase-locked action potentials; the afferents form large club terminals on large spherical cells which have few or no dendrites and thick axons. The spherical cells form no local connections within the lateral line lobe, but relay timing information directly to the midbrain torus. The lateral line lobe is divided into multiple somatotopically organized zones. It was a mystery as to why different zones might have the same sensory input until anatomical and physiological studies demonstrated that the 3 maps differed in the size of their afferent terminal fields, and in the temporal and spatial frequency of the responses of their cells. The parallel processing of electrosensory information in each map appears to be adapted to detect objects of varying spatial frequency [38].

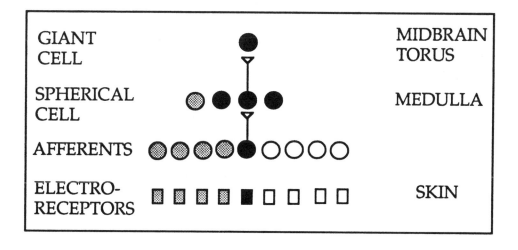

Fig. 2. *Schematic circuit for encoding phase information that impinges on the body surface. Between 3-4 phase-coding electroreceptors converge on spherical cells in the medulla (stippled cells) that in turn converge in a topographic projection onto giant cells in the torus (filled cells). Each torus cell receives convergent inputs from between 3-4 spherical cells and therefore 9-16 afferents.* [7,12].

Time coding improves with the progression from receptors to primary afferents to spherical cells to giant cells in the midbrain torus [3]. The accuracy of the phase-coding was determined by measuring action potentials from phase coders in the medulla and in the midbrain torus. The jitter of these action potentials, defined as the standard deviation of the response time to the stimulus, decreased three-fold with the progression from medulla to midbrain. The basis for this improvement of accuracy may lie in the convergence from afferents to higher level neurons. Afferents converge upon spherical cells which converge on giant cells in the torus (Fig. 2). These convergent inputs from phase-coding afferents should reduce the jitter by /N of the number of inputs, or 3-4 times. This predicted improvement in jitter is close to the measured decrease in jitter from 30 μs in the medulla to 10 μs in the midbrain. Since the accuracy of even the best single neurons in these first stations of the time coding pathway does not match that of the behavior [3,33], electric fish are said to display temporal hyperacuity or reliable discrimination of microsecond time differences. Because their temporal resolution is far superior to that observed in the primary electrosensory afferents, and is far shorter than the duration of the action potential, this hyperacuity must result from extensive parallel computations and network processing.

3.2   The Auditory System

The behavioral experiments described in section 2.2 showed that most animals use interaural phase differences to localize sound. Time coding must originate at the level of the sensory cell, although there are as yet few studies on how the auditory hair cell transduction process encodes and retains the phase structure of the stimulus. The modulating signal at the spike generator in the primary afferent auditory nerve fiber arises from components of the hair cell receptor potential, via a chemical synapse [48].

The extent of phase-locking to the stimulus is quantified by the vector strength [9] (Fig. 3). Vector strength decreases with increasing frequency, and these decreases have been interpreted as showing that the neurons's ability to phase-lock decreases with frequency [48]. Recordings from auditory nerve fibers have shown that action potentials phase-lock to the waveform of the acoustic stimulus [19]. Spikes occur most frequently at a particular phase of the tone, although not necessarily in every tonal cycle. Thus the discharge pattern of a cochlear nerve fiber can encode the phase of a tone with a frequency above 1000 Hz even though the average discharge rate is low.

Auditory hair cells encode and transmit both phase and amplitude information to the auditory nerve. Since these primary afferents phase-lock to the auditory stimulus, and encode amplitude by increases in spike rate, there can be no separate coding of amplitude or phase in the periphery, unlike electric fish. The same parallel

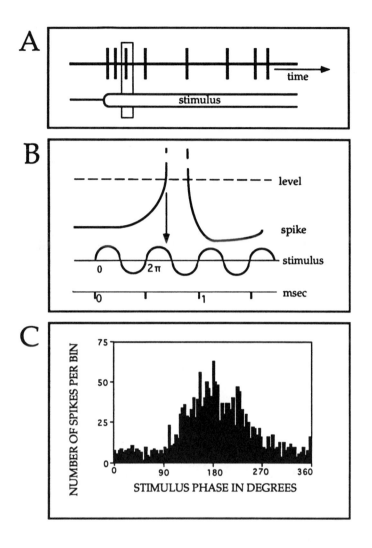

Fig. 3: A. *Timing information is encoded by phase-locked action potentials.* B. *Spike timing is measured with respect to the phase of the stimulus.* C. *Spike phase is plotted in a period histogram which is used to calculate vector strength (r). The distribution of phase angles in the period histogram is measured; if most action potentials fall within a small range of phase angles, the vector strength is high (near 1) and if action potentials are evenly distributed, the vector strength is near 0. Vector strength is determined as follows: Each spike defines a vector of unit length with a phase angle θ. The x and y components of the vector are x=cos θ and y=sin θ. The n vectors characterizing the action potentials are plotted on a unit circle and the mean vector calulated as θ= arctan ($\Sigma y/\Sigma x$) + $k\pi$, where k=0 or 1 depending on the signs of Σy and Σx. The length of the mean vector, r = $\sqrt{(\Sigma x)^2 + (\Sigma y)^2}/n$, provides a measure of the degree of synchronization.*

processing of phase and amplitude information that characterizes the electrosensory system is, however also found in the auditory system. Although the segregation into two channnels does not begin at the level of the receptors, differences in auditory nerve terminals creates a similar functional segregation in the central nervous system. Auditory nerve afferents enter the brain and divide into two branches, one which ramifies in the dendritic field of the amplitude coding cochlear nucleus angularis, while the other branch terminates in the phase-coding cochlear nucleus magnocellularis [46]. The terminal in the nucleus magnocellularis forms a specialized ending termed an endbulb of Held [1,35]. The endbulb synapse conveys the phase-locked discharge of the auditory nerve fibers to their postsynaptic targets in the nucleus magnocellularis. Thus the synaptic specializations in the auditory nerve accomplish the same goal as the receptor specialization in electric fish.

Auditory hair cells encode and transmit both phase and amplitude information to the auditory nerve. Since these primary afferents phase-lock to the auditory stimulus, and encode amplitude by increases in spike rate, there can be no separate coding of amplitude or phase in the periphery, unlike electric fish. The same parallel processing of phase and amplitude information that characterizes the electrosensory system is, however also found in the auditory system. Although the segregation into two channnels does not begin at the level of the receptors, differences in auditory nerve terminals creates a similar functional segregation in the central nervous system. Auditory nerve afferents enter the brain and divide into two branches, one which ramifies in the dendritic field of the amplitude coding cochlear nucleus angularis, while the other branch terminates in the phase-coding cochlear nucleus magnocellularis [46]. The terminal in the nucleus magnocellularis forms a specialized ending termed an endbulb of Held [1,35]. The endbulb synapse conveys the phase-locked discharge of the auditory nerve fibers to their postsynaptic targets in the nucleus magnocellularis. Thus the synaptic specializations in the auditory nerve accomplish the same goal as the receptor specialization in electric fish.

The endbulb is specialized to preserve phase-locked signals (Fig. 4). Each endbulb has multiple sites of synaptic contact on the soma to provide the substrate for the preservation of the phase-locked action potentials between the auditory nerve fibers and the neurons of the nucleus magnocellularis. The endbulb is a secure and effective connection; physiological measures show that phase-locking is the same or better in the neurons of the nucleus magnocellularis than in the eighth nerve, while it is lost in the projection to the amplitude coding nucleus angularis. There are also specializations at the receptor level; magnocellular neurons in barn owl and chick have fast synaptic potentials [10], and a recent study of chick magnocellular neurons has shown that stimulation of glutamate receptors produces large currents with unusually fast onset and termination [32].

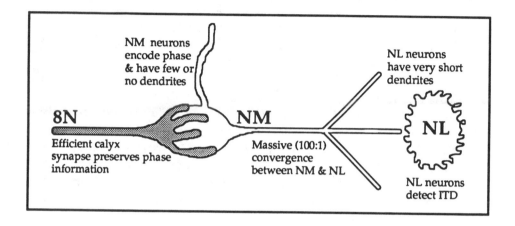

Fig. 4: *The auditory nerve (8N) forms endbulb terminals on nucleus magnocellularis (NM) neurons. These cells project to the neurons of the nucleus laminaris (NL).*

The auditory system uses phase-locked signals for the measurement of time disparities. Phase information is preserved and improved, and interaural phase differences are detected, in a circuit composed of the cochlear nucleus magnocellularis and the nucleus laminaris (Fig. 4). Many of the features of this circuit appear to be associated with the encoding of timing information. Magnocellular neurons have large round cell bodies, a thick axon and few medium length dendrites [17]. In the owl, magnocellular neurons in the high best frequency regions of the nucleus have fewer dendrites than the neurons in the low best frequency region [4]. These reductions in dendritic area would decrease the input resistance of the cell, decrease the membrane time constant and improve the speed and accuracy of the phase-locked response to synaptic inputs.

The nucleus magnocellularis relays phase-locked action potentials in a bilateral projection to the nucleus laminaris. There is a further improvement in phase-locking between the nucleus magnocellularis and the nucleus laminaris [6]. The improved phase locking may be caused in part by the convergence of magnocellular afferents onto laminaris neurons, since about 100 inputs from each nucleus magnocellularis converge on each laminaris neuron. Furthermore, laminaris neurons have very short dendrites, which should be isopotential with the cell body. These cells should therefore, like magnocellular neurons, have accurate and fast responses to phase-locked inputs (Fig. 4).

4   Detecting time differences

Behavioral experiments have shown great accuracy in detecting time differences. Detection of time differences was first modelled by Jeffress in his place theory [16]. The model circuit is composed of two elements, *delay lines* and *coincidence detectors*   (Fig. 5). The delay lines are created by axons of varying length, and the coincidence detectors are neurons that respond maximally when they receive simultaneous inputs, i.e. when the time difference is exactly compensated for by the delay introduced by the inputs.

Circuits in the fish midbrain, the auditory brainstem of barn owls, cats and dogs, and the bat thalamus all contain neurons tuned to particular time delays between events. These delay-tuned ensembles employ similar algorithms. The circuits in the auditory brainstem resemble the Jeffress model, while the circuits in fish midbrain and bat thalamus differ from the Jeffress model in significant respects. The circuit in the fish midbrain does not form a place map, while the circuits in the bat thalamus seem not use axonal delay lines, but synaptic delays instead.

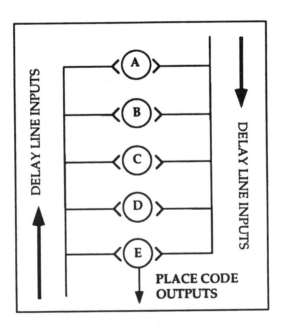

Fig. 5 *Jeffress model with coincidence detectors A-E and delay line inputs from each channel. Note that the position or place of each coincidence detector dictates its preferred time difference.*

4.1   Detection of Phase Differences in Electric Fish

Weakly electric fish can distinguish phase differences as small as 0.5 μs between different parts of the body surface. The circuit for detection of these phase differences is composed of phase-coding afferents from the medulla which project to two cell types of the midbrain torus. The medullary phase coders synapse on giant cell bodies and on the dendrites of the small cells (Fig. 6). The inputs to the small cell dendrites encode the phase of the electric organ discharge from one part of body surface. The giant cell's axons form horizontal connections that distribute this local phase information to small cells throughout the lamina, so that timing information from one part of the body surface may be compared with any other part. Small cells compare information from differents parts of the body surface [14]. This circuit allows the fish to perform all possible comparisons between different parts of the body surface, as required for correct performance of the jamming avoidance response.

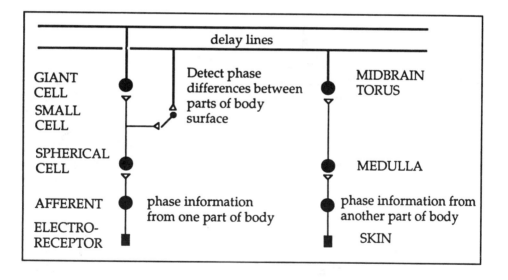

Fig. 6: *Schematic circuit in the electric fish midbrain for computation of phase differences between signals on any two parts of the body surface. Electrosensory information converges in a topographic projection onto giant cell bodies and small cell dendrites in the torus. Giant cells relay the phase-locked signal all over the torus, with their terminals synapsing on the cell bodies of small cells. Small cells are therefore able to compare phase information from different parts of the body surface [7,12].*

The phase sensitivity of the small cells is less than that of the behavior. Although the temporal acuity of single neurons improves at each level of the time coding pathway, the smallest temporal disparity detected by the most sensitive neurons in the torus is only 10 µs, a value 20x higher that the behavioral threshold [3]. If the responses of such neurons are averaged over periods that are much longer than the 300 ms latency of the jamming avoidance response, a sensitivity to 1 µs can be demonstrated [33]. Since the temporal averaging of the electrophysiologist is assumed to be equivalent to spatial averaging or parallel processing of the same signal in the CNS, this suggests that the sensitivity and short latency of the jamming avoidance response requires parallel convergence of large numbers of such toral neurons, carrying temporal information from wide areas of the body surface [33]. This convergence ultimately occurs at the level of single neurons in the pre-pacemaker nucleus [18]. Sensitivity to small temporal disparities does exist at the single neuron level [18]. Neurons in the prepacemaker nucleus regulate the frequency of the fish's electric organ discharge, and modulate their firing with changes in the interfering signal, even with temporal disparities as small as 1 µs [18]. Thus the hyperacuity may be achieved by a network of prepacemaker neurons.

4.2   Detection of Interaural Phase Differences in the Barn Owl

Detection of interaural time differences in the nucleus laminaris depends upon coincidence detection and delay lines as outlined in the Jeffress (1948) model. The Jeffress model explains not only how interaural time differences are measured but also how they are encoded. The circuit contains an array of coincidence detectors receiving input from afferent axons serving as delay lines. Because of its position in the array, each neuron responds only to sound coming from a particular direction, and thus the anatomical place of the neuron encodes the location of the sound (Fig. 7). These neurons use the temporal information to compute a new variable, time difference, and transform the time code into a place code. The selectivity of all higher-order auditory neurons to time difference derives from the"labelled-line" output of the place map (Konishi, 1986).

The circuit in the barn owl's auditory brainstem that detects interaural phase differences resembles the Jeffress model. The cochlear nucleus axons act as delay lines, and the laminaris neurons act as coincidence detectors, to form a circuit that measures and encodes interaural time differences (Fig. 7). Early physiological studies of the mammalian auditory system by Goldberg and Brown (1969) and others found neuronal responses consistent with the Jeffress model, and recent results in the barn owl [6,43], cat [39,49] and chicken [30,34,50] have described circuits that conform to the model's requirements. The Jeffress model has three major parts: delay lines, coincidence detection and place coding of interaural phase difference.

In the barn owl, magnocellular axons act as delay lines [5,6]. The axons convey the timing or phase of the auditory stimulus in a bilateral projection to the nucleus laminaris such that axons from the ipsilateral nucleus magnocellularis enter the nucleus laminaris from the dorsal side, while axons from the contralateral nucleus magnocellularis enter from the ventral side. Thus these afferents interdigitate to innervate dorso-ventral arrays of neurons in laminaris in a sequential fashion (Fig. 7). Recordings from these interdigitating ipsilateral and contralateral axons show regular changes in delay with depth in the nucleus laminaris [15]. These conduction delays are similar to the 200 μs range of interaural time differences available to the barn owl [26]. The conduction velocities of the delay lines may be regulated by the internodal distances within the nucleus laminaris. Normal internode lengths in the central nervous system are generally greater than 300 μm [47], while internode lengths in the delay lines axons in the nucleus laminaris are both short and regular, occurring every 60 μm [15].

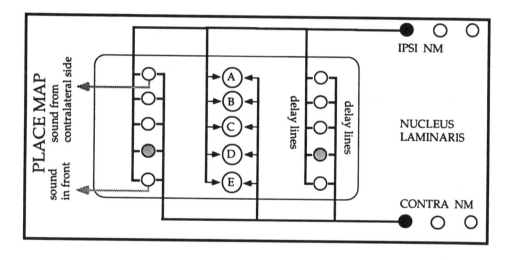

Fig. 7 *Jeffress model and schematic of brainstem auditory circuits for detection of interaural time differences in the barn owl. Axons from the ipsilateral cochlear nucleus magnocellularis (IPSI NM) divide and enter the nucleus laminaris at several points along the dorsal surface. These axons act as delay lines within laminaris, interdigitating with inputs from the contralateral cochlear nucleus magnocellularis (CONTRA NM). Coincidence detectors A-E fire maximally when inputs from the two sides arrive simultaneously. This can only occur when the interaural phase differences are compensated for by an equal and opposite delay. Thus this array forms a map of interaural time difference in the dorso-ventral dimension of the nucleus. In the owl, sound from the front is mapped towards the ventral surface of the nucleus, and each nucleus contains place maps of the contralateral and part of the ipsilateral hemifield [modified from [21]].*

A major requirement of the Jeffress model is that the targets of the delay lines act as coincidence detectors. Goldberg & Brown [9] showed that olivary neurons acted as coincidence detectors. The neurons of the nucleus laminaris and the medial superior olive phase-lock to both monaural and binaural stimuli, and they respond maximally when phase-locked spikes from each side arrive simultaneously, i.e. when the difference in the internal conduction delay is nullified by interaural time difference. The number of spikes elicited in response to a favorable interaural time difference is roughly double that elicited by a monaural stimulus, while spike counts for unfavorable interaural time differences fall well below monaural response levels. Thus, physiological responses from these coincidence detectors are similar [6,9,42,49].

5   Summary and Conclusions

Time coding is prominent in both the electrosensory and auditory systems. Both systems use similar algorithms where phase-locked action potentials encode the timing of the stimulus, and the CNS uses this code for the measurement of time disparities. Time and amplitude information is processed in parallel. Phase-coding improves with convergence from the periphery to higher level processing stations. The morphology and physiology of phase-coding cells is suited to their function; they have large cell bodies with few or no dendrites, thick axons and short duration action potentials.

5.1   Comparisons with other vertebrate systems

There are a number of other systems which have been shown to employ delay lines and coincidence detectors to compute relevant features of the stimulus. There is not a great deal of information about the characteristics of concidence detectors, but delays may be encoded and processed in the central nervous system in a number of ways. One example is found in echolocating bats. These animals emit orientation sounds and listen to the returning echos. The delay between the pulse and echo conveys the target distance [40]. The echo delay is therefore a behaviorally relevant stimulus. Echo delay is not encoded at the periphery, where neurons respond to the pulse and the echo, and the time interval between the two grouped discharges is directly related to the echo delay. At higher levels of the auditory system, however, neurons are found which respond strongly when pulse and echo are combined with a particular echo delay. These "combination-sensitive" neurons were first found in the auditory cortex of the mustache bat, where echo-delay is mapped on the cortical surface to form maps of target range [28,41]. In order for the echo evoked activity to coincide with the pulse, the pulse signal must be delayed with reference to the echo. The generation of delays is more complex than that in the auditory brainstem because of the time delays (0.5-20 ms) are very much larger than the 200 µs interaural time differences available to the barn owl [6] or 400 µs for the cat [49]. Two other mechanisms may be used for delaying the pulse signal. For best delays below 4 ms, delay tuning depends only on coincidence of pulse and echo excitation. This result is consistent with delay lines created by excitatory relay units. For long best delays (> 4 ms), the FM1 pulse produces inhibition of short latency and variable duration, followed by excitation, consistent with the "inhibitory gate" hypothesis [44] in which FM1 delays are created by varying the duration of inhibition. The inhibition may be produced by local circuits within the medial geniculate body [29].

Similar observations have been made in the visual thalamus. In the lateral geniculate, inhibition produces the X-lagged cell responses [24,25]. These geniculate cells differ from their retinal X-afferent inputs and from adjacent non-lagged geniculate X-cells in displaying an early inhibition rather excitation to the onset of a visual stimulus in their receptive field. The X-lagged response is delayed because the excitatory input is blocked by inhibition, not because excitation is delayed. Postinhibitory rebound then produces the lagged or phase-shifted response. The response timing differences between lagged and nonlagged cells may be important for directing direction selectivity in visual cortex [36]. These observations also reflect the pioneering theoretical and physiological observations from the Reichart group in Tubingen on motion sensitivity in the insect visual system [32a]. The Reichart model of directional selectivity in the visual system connected two detectors to an AND-NOT gate, one via a delay (reviewed in Marr, 1982).

Time coding systems implement similar algorithms for the measurement of time differences. These algorithms all depend on delay lines and coincidence detectors in some form. Short delays may be provided by axonal delay lines. Axons have been known to provide functionally significant delays in conduction, and compensatory delay line mechanisms include equalization of path length, differences in conduction velocity and localized delays, determined by variations in preterminal axon branches [47]. Long delays may be introduced by interposed excitatory synapses, while the longest delays originate with inhibitory interneurons and regulation of post-inhibitory rebound. Neural circuits that incorporate delays may be widespread in the CNS. The underlying mechanism(s) of the recipient coincidence detection are less well understood than those that generate delays. It is clear, however, that the coincidence detectors use the time code to detect inputs within some particular time window and that they then transform these signals into perceptions such as sound location or target range.

5.2   Conclusions

Analysis of the encoding and processing of temporal information has uncovered some common organizational principles. Time coding systems implement similar algorithms for the encoding and processing of temporal information [21]. Despite different neural substrates, the CNS time channels share numerous morphological and physiological adaptations to improve the time-coding of signal. In most senses, including the electric sense, audition and vision, coding for the timing or phase of the signal and coding for its amplitude are carried out in parallel. In electric fish, parallel processing of phase and amplitude begins at the receptor level, while in the auditory system the separation into phase and amplitude coding is derived within the central nervous system. The separation of visual information into two channels which differ in their spatial and temporal acuity begins in the retina [22].

6   References

[1]   Brawer, J.R. and Morest, D.K.: Relations between auditory nerve endings and cell types in the cat's anteroventral cochlear nucleus seen with Golgi method and Nomarski optics, J. Comp. Neurol., **160**, pp.491-506 (1974).

[2]   Bullock, T.H., Hamstra, R.H. and Scheich, H.: The jamming avoidance response of high frequency electric fish. I. General features, J. Comp. Physiol., **77**, pp.1-22 (1972).

[3]   Carr, C., Heiligenberg, W. and Rose, G.: A time-comparison circuit in the electric fish midbrain. I. Behavior and physiology, J. Neurosci., **6**, pp.107-119 (1986).

[4]   Carr, C.E. and Boudreau, R.E.: Organization of the nucleus magnocellularis and the nucleus laminaris in the barn owl: encoding and measuring interaural time differences, J. Comp. Neurol., **334**, pp. 337-355 (1992)

[5]   Carr, C.E. and Konishi, M.: Axonal delay lines for time measurement in the owl's brainstem, Proc. Natl. Acad. Sci., **85**, pp.8311-8315 (1988).

[6]   Carr, C.E. and Konishi, M.: A circuit for detection of interaural time differences in the brainstem of the barn owl, J. Neurosci., **10**, pp.3227-3246 (1990).

[7]   Carr, C.E., Maler, L. and Taylor, B.: A time comparison circuit in the electric fish midbrain. II. Functional morphology, J. Neurosci., **6**, pp.1372-1383 (1986).

[8]   Fay, R.R., *Hearing in vertebrates: A psychophysics databook*, Hill-Fay Associates, Winnetka, Illinois, 1988,

[9]   Goldberg, J.M. and Brown, P.B.: Response of binaural neurons of dog superior olivary complex to dichotic tonal stimuli: Some physiological mechanisms of sound localization, J. Neurophysiol., **32**, pp.613-636 (1969).

[10]   Hackett, J.T. and Rubel, E.W.: Synaptic excitation of the second and third order auditory neurons in the avian brain stem, Neurosci., **7**, pp.1455-1469 (1982).

[11] Heffner, R.S. and Heffner, H.E., Evolution of sound localization in mammals. In D.B. Webster, R.R. Fay and A.N. Popper (Eds.), *The evolutionary biology of hearing*, Springer-Verlag, New York, 1992, pp. 691-716.

[12] Heiligenberg, W., *Neural nets in electric fish*, MIT Press, Cambridge, Massachusetts, 1991,

[13] Heiligenberg, W., Baker, C. and Matsubara, J.A.: The jamming avoidance response in Eigenmannia revisited: The structure of a neuronal democracy, J. Comp. Physiol., **127**, pp.267-286 (1978).

[14] Heiligenberg, W. and Rose, G.: Phase and amplitude computations in the midbrain of an electric fish: intracellular studies of neurons participating in the jamming avoidance response of Eigenmannia, J. Neurosci., **5**, pp.515-531 (1985).

[15] Heiligenberg, W. and Rose, G.J.: The optic tectum of the gymnotiform electric fish, Eigenmannia, labeling of physiologically identified cells, Neurosci., **22**, pp.331-340 (1987).

[16] Jeffress, L.A.: A place theory of sound localization, J. Comp. Physiol. Psych., **41**, pp.35-39 (1948).

[17] Jhaveri, S. and Morest, K.: Neuronal architecture in nucleus magnocellularis of the chicken auditory system with observations on nucleus laminaris: A light and electron microscope study, Neurosci., **7**, pp.809-836 (1982).

[18] Kawasaki, M., Rose, G. and Heiligenberg, W.: Temporal hyperacuity in single neurons of electric fish, Nature, **336**, pp.173-176 (1988).

[19] Kiang, N.Y.S., Watanabe, T., Thomas, E.C. and Clark, E.F., *Discharge patterns of single fibers in the cat's auditory nerve*, MIT Press, Cambridge, Massachusetts, 1965,

[20] Konishi, M.: How the owl tracks its prey, Am. Sci., **61**, pp.414-424 (1973)

[21] Konishi, M.: Deciphering the brain's codes, Neural Computation, **3**, pp.1-18 (1991).

[22] Livingstone, M.L. and Hubel, D.H.: Psychophysical evidence for separate channels for the perception of form, color, movement and depth, J. Neurosci., **7**, pp.3416-3468 (1987).

[23] Masters, W.M., Moffat, A.J.M. and Simmons, J.A.: Sonar tracking of horizontally moving targets by the big brown bat Eptesicus fuscus, Science, **228**, pp.1331-1333 (1985).

[24] Mastronade, D.N.: Two classes of single-input X-cells in cat lateral geniculate nucleus. I. Receptive field properties and classification of cells, J. Neurophysiol., **57**, pp.357-380 (1987).

[25] Mastronade, D.N.: Two classes of single input cell in the lateral geniculate nucleus. II. Retinal inputs and the generation of receptive field properties, J. Neurophysiol., **57**, pp.381-413 (1987).

[26] Moiseff, A.: Binaural disparity cues available to the barn owl for sound localization, J. Comp. Physiol., **164**, pp.629-636 (1989).

[27]   Moiseff, A. and Konishi, M.: Neuronal and Behavioral Sensitivity to Binaural Time Differences in the Owl, J. Neurosci., 1, pp.40-48 (1981).

[28]   O'Neill, W.E. and Suga, N.: Encoding of target range information and its representation in the auditory cortex of the mustache bat, J. Neurosci., 2, pp.17-31 (1982).

[29]   Olsen, J.F.j and Suga, N.: Combination-Sensitive Neurons in the Medial Geniculate Body of the Mustached Bat: Encoding of Target Range Information, J. Neurophysiol., 65, pp.1275 (1991).

[30]   Overholt, T., Hyson, R. and Rubel, E.W.: A delay-line circuit for coding interaural time differences in the chick brain stem, J. Neurosci., (1992)

[31]   Payne, R.S.: Acoustic localization of prey by barn owls (Tyto alba), J. Exp. Biol., 54, pp.535-573 (1971).

[32]   Raman, I. and Trussell, L.O.: The kinetics of the responses to glutamate and kainate in neurons of the avian cochlear nucleus, Neuron, 9, pp.173-186 (1992).

[32a] Reichardt, W. and Poggio, T. Visual control of orientation behavior in the fly. Part 1. A quantitative analysis, Quart. Rev. Biophys. 9, 311-375 (1976).

[33]   Rose, G. and Heiligenberg, W.: Temporal hyperacuity in the electric sense of fish, Nature, 318, pp.178-180 (1985).

[34]   Rubel, E.W. and Parks, T.N.: Organization and Development of Brain Stem Auditory Nuclei of the Chicken:]Tonotopic Organization of N. magnocellularis and N. laminaris, J. Comp. Neurol., 164, pp.411-434 (1975).

[35]   Ryugo, D.K. and Fekete, D.M.: Morphology of primary axosomatic endings in the anteroventral cochlear nucleus of the cat: A study of the endbulbs of Held, J. Comp. Neurol., 210, pp.239-257 (1982).

[36]   Saul, A.B. and Humphrey, A.L.: Spatial and temporal response properties of lagged and non-lagged cells in cat lateral geniculate nucleus, J. Neurophysiol., 64, pp.206-224 (1990).

[37]   Scheich, H., Bullock, T.H. and Hamstra, R.H.: Coding properties of two classes of afferent nerve fibers: High frequency electroreceptors in the electric fish Eigenmannia, J. Neurophysiol., 36, pp.39-60 (1973).

[38]   Shumway, C.A.: Multiple electrosensory maps in the medulla of weakly electric Gymnotiform fish. I. Physiological differences, J. Neurosci., 9, pp.-32768 (1989).

[39]   Smith, P.H., Joris, P.X. and Yin, T.C.T., Projections of physiologically characterized spherical bushy cell axons from the cochlear nucleus of the cat: evidence for delay lines to the medial superior olive, J. Comp. Neurol, in press (1993).

[40]   Suga, N.: Cortical computational maps for auditory imaging, Neural Networks, 3, pp.3-21 (1990).

[41]   Suga, N., O'Neill, W.E. and Manabe, T.: Cortical neurons sensitive to combinations of information bearing elements of biosonar signals in the mustache bat, Science, **200**, pp.778-781 (1978).

[42]   Sullivan, W.E and Konishi, M.: Segregation of stimulus phase and intensity coding in the cochlear nucleus of the barn owl, J. Neurosci., **4**, pp.1787-1799 (1984).

[43]   Sullivan, W.E and Konishi, M.: Neural map of interaural phase difference in the owl's brainstem, Proc. Natl. Acad. Sci., **83**, pp.8400-8404 (1986).

[44]   Sullivan, W.E.: Possible neural mechanisms of target distance coding in auditory system of the echolocating bat Myotis lucifugis, J. Neurophysiol., **48**, pp.1033-1047 (1982).

[45]   Szabo, T.: Sense Organs of the Lateral Line System in some Electric Fish of the Gymnotidae, Mormyridae and Gynmarchidae, Journal of Morphology, **117**, pp.229-250 (1965).

[46]   Takahashi, T., Moiseff, A. and Konishi, M.: Time and intensity cues are processed independently in the auditory system of the owl, J. Neurosci., **4**, pp.1781-1786 (1984).

[47]   Waxman, S.G.: Integrative properties and design principles of axons, Int. Rev. Neurobiol., **18**, pp.1-40 (1975).

[48]   Weiss, T.F. and Rose, C.: A comparison of synchronization filters in different auditory receptor organs, Hear. Res., **33**, pp.175-180 (1988).

[49]   Yin, T.C.T. and Chan, J.C.K.: Interaural time sensitivity in medial superior olive of cat, J. Neurophysiol., **64**, pp.465-488 (1990).

[50]   Young, S.R. and Rubel, E.W.: Frequency-specific projections of individual neurons in chick brainstem auditory nuclei, J. Neurosci., **7**, pp.1373-1378 (1983).

Chapter 2
Adaptive Movement Computation By The Blowfly Visual System *

R.R. de Ruyter van Steveninck [†]   W. Bialek [†]   M.Potters [‡§]

R.H. Carlson [‡]   G.D. Lewen [†]

Abstract

We consider the problem of visually estimating wide-field rigid motion in the presence of noise. Biologically this is a highly relevant problem, because motion estimation is important in animal navigation and course stabilization. It is therefore presumably beneficial for the animal to use the information gathered by the photoreceptors in a statistically optimal way. A theoretical analysis of the problem shows that the optimal processor should adapt its computational strategy to the statistics of the environment. In this paper we present experimental evidence indicating the blowfly's brain tries to adapt its strategy of movement computation in a way consistent with the theoretical results.

1   Introduction

Here we combine ideas from two lines of research in visual information processing. The first is the study of the fundamental limits to the reliability of selected visual tasks as set by noise at the photoreceptor level. The second is the attempt to describe certain important visual tasks in a functional mathematical framework. Probably the clearest example of the latter approach can be found in the work of Reichardt and collaborators. Starting with a formulation for the fundamental interactions involved in movement detection [18], see also Sect. 2, this line of thought was generalized to more complex visual computations, such as figure-ground discrimination [20], and given a systematic mathematical formulation in terms of Volterra

---

*Based on, and substantially updated from, "Statistical adaptation and optimal estimation in movement computation by the blowfly visual system" by R.R. de Ruyter van Steveninck, W. Bialek, M. Potters, R.H. Carlson which appeared in IEEE International Conference on Systems, Man and Cybernetics; Oct 2-5, 1994, San Antonio, TX; pp. 302-307. ©1994 IEEE.

[†]NEC Research Institute, 4 Independence Way, Princeton NJ 08540

[‡]Department of Physics, Princeton University

[§]present address: Universita di Roma, Rome Italy

series by Poggio and Reichardt [15]. These authors have always emphasized the fundamental role played by nonlinear interactions in solving nontrivial visual tasks.

Early examples of the first line of research are Hecht et al. [10] and van der Velden [31], who were interested in questions pertaining to the detectability of single photons, and in de Vries [30] and Rose [21] who analyzed the effects of photon shot noise on simple perceptual tasks. The work in this field was extended to measuring the reliability of nerve responses [1]. Research into factors limiting the accuracy of vision has been very productive, and over the years the results have lent more support to the notion that visual signal processing may approach optimal performance under the right conditions [29]. Generally speaking, however, this line of research has been constrained to relatively simple stimuli where the total energy could be well-defined, such as light flashes, presentations of gratings for limited intervals and the like. The detection task in such cases ultimately consists of estimating a (positive or negative) excess photon count over a linearly weighted area of the retina. Although we certainly gain insight into the statistical efficiency of various processing levels in the visual system, many interesting higher visual functions are not probed in this way. To our knowledge, the case of nonlinear interactions between noisy photoreceptor signals has received little attention. In the following we therefore revisit the problem of a well-defined nonlinear computation, namely movement detection. But instead of assuming noiseless input as in Reichardt's original approach, we will explicitly incorporate noise in the photoreceptors that provide the input to the computation. For simple movement stimuli such as sudden displacement steps of wide field patterns, this problem is tractable. Comparing measurements of the statistical efficiency of the blowfly movement-sensitive neuron known as H1 with the performance of an ideal observer who uses realistic photoreceptor signals [26], we find that over a 10 ms time interval the neuron approaches the ideal observer closely. It thus seems that under these simple conditions, the fly tries to compute movement in an optimal way on a behaviorally relevant time scale. One of the questions prompted by this result is whether optimal processing can be generalized to more complex visual tasks, and if so, what role adaptational processes may play in this.

2 Visual information processing; models for movement detection

Visual information processing begins with a spatially ordered mapping of light intensities in the environment onto the retina. The retina essentially consists of an array of photoreceptor cells that convert the light intensities they receive into electrical signals. Introspectively it seems that our percepts are generated without any effort at all. In reality, however, the brain is constantly carrying out computations on the signals provided by its sense organs to extract useful information from them. This computational task is generally far from simple. Consider for example the complexity of the signals in the array of photoreceptors as the animal moves through a highly complex and variable three-dimensional environment which may contain other moving objects as well. Furthermore, there are physical limitations to the incoming signal due to diffraction and to the random arrival of photons. The statistical structure of the signals in the photoreceptor array is therefore very complicated, and one of the motivations for experimental work on sensory information processing is our sheer lack of understanding of how, even in principle, many of the brain's computational tasks can be solved.

As light intensities in the environment vary over a wide range, so will the signal to noise ratio of the photoreceptor signals. To accommodate the variation in light flux, photoreceptors are highly adaptive in their gain and dynamics. Fly photoreceptors seem designed to operate close (i.e. within a factor two or three) to the limits imposed by photon flux, up to at least $3 \cdot 10^5$ photoconversions per second [28]. As it is metabolically expensive to sustain these rates of photoconversion, it seems plausible that the brain of a well-designed fly tries to use this hard-won information to the fullest. Indeed, we find that in a simple movement discrimination task, the fly's brain is able to use a substantial amount of the total information present in the photoreceptor array [26, 27]. Inspired by this and by the observation of adaptation in the peripheral visual system, we explore some questions relating to the problem of adaptive computation on input signals corrupted by noise.

To examine this experimentally, we record responses from a wide-field movement sensitive cell, classified as H1, in the lobula plate of the blowfly's brain. For our goal, this cell has a few distinct advantages. First of all, and this is relatively rare in neurophysiology, we have a good idea of its function. Through a combination of anatomical, physiological and behavioural studies [14, 7, 8, 9] it has become clear that H1 and other wide-field cells in the lobula plate collect movement information over large visual fields and send this information to the thoracic ganglion. There these signals are used as inputs to the motor control system responsible for maintaining stable flight. For this purpose the fly is presumably mainly interested in estimating self motion, especially rotation, and less in sensing motions of other objects. The second advantage is that movement detection can only be accomplished by a nonlinear operation on the array of photoreceptor signals [15], which makes it very interesting from the point of view of the propagation of input noise into the final result. Third, the basic operation is relatively simple, so that we can hope to obtain some analytical results.

In the literature a distinction is made between two types of biological movement detectors. The oldest one, the correlator model formulated by Reichardt [18, 19] is based on a correlation between a delayed signal from one

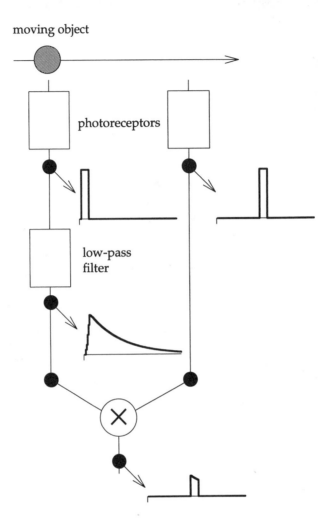

FIG. 1. *Simplified version of a Reichardt movement detector. When an object moves across the visual field, it induces a brief electrical response in one photoreceptor and a similar response in a neighboring receptor somewhat later. The response of one photoreceptor is fed into a low-pass filter having an impulse response with a long tail. The output of this filter and the output of the second photoreceptor are multiplied to produce an output with a pulse height depending on the velocity of movement. As can be seen, the response depends on other parameters as well, such as the contrast of the object.*

direction of view with a direct signal from a neighboring direction. A simple realization is depicted in Fig. 1. As the basic principle of operation consists of correlating linearly filtered photoreceptor signals, it is immediately clear that the model provides an ambiguous readout of velocity. For example, the model's output is proportional to the square of the contrast of a moving pattern. In addition, the response depends on spatial details of the pattern. An alternative was formulated by Limb and Murphy [11]. In principle their model takes the ratio of the time and space derivatives of a rigidly moving pattern. In other words:

$$(1) \qquad \vec{v}_{est}(t) = -\frac{\nabla_t I(\vec{r}(t))}{\nabla_{\vec{r}} I(\vec{r}(t))},$$

where $I(\vec{r}(t))$ is the pattern's light intensity in space and time. For a pattern moving at velocity $\vec{v}(t)$ we have:

$$(2) \qquad \vec{v}_{est}(t) = -\frac{I' \cdot d\vec{r}(t)/dt}{I'} = \vec{v}(t),$$

and the model computes velocity, independent of other stimulus parameters. In the literature, experimental support can be found for both these models over a range of animals from insects to humans [13].

Both models were formulated in a somewhat ad-hoc fashion, and neither model takes the effects of input noise into account. In the following we address the question of movement detection on a first-principles basis. The guiding principle is the desideratum to make the most accurate least-squares estimate of the velocity of a wide-field pattern, given the signal-to-noise characteristics of the photoreceptors. This is in line with what we know about the function of H1 in the fly's brain. The full mathematical treatment is beyond the scope of this paper, but can be found elsewhere [3, 16, 17]. Instead we present a more intuitive approach which can be understood from first principles. Some of the predictions are presented and compared to experimental findings.

One implication is that qualitative aspects of the computation should change when the signal-to-noise ratio (SNR) at the photoreceptor level changes from a high to a low value. A rather dramatic demonstration of this is the prediction that the optimal velocity estimator should approach the gradient scheme [11] at high SNR, because this gives a velocity estimate without systematic error. However, at low SNR, this leads to disastrous results, because of the noisy term in the denominator of Eq. 1. At low SNR the velocity estimator should shift its computation to a form of the original Reichardt correlator, with a multiplicative interaction between two linearly filtered versions of the photoreceptor signals. This is forced by a tradeoff between statistical and systematic errors: At high SNR, the optimal estimator can afford to compute high-order terms between photoreceptor signals, thus improving its velocity estimate by reducing systematic error.

At low SNR, however, the statistical error in higher order terms in the computation grows faster than in lower order terms. Therefore, at very low SNR only the lowest-order term that contains any movement information, i.e. the quadratic one, should be used.

The transition between the two regimes is smooth, and the particular version of the gradient model predicted can be seen as a suitably normalized version of a Reichardt correlator, where the normalization adapts to the SNR. A simplified version of this adaptive movement sensor can be derived for a case in which the image motion is diffusive, and characterized by a diffusion constant D. Then the optimal estimator should compute:

$$(3) \qquad \vec{v}_{est}(t) \approx -\frac{\int d\vec{r}\, \nabla_{\vec{r}} S \cdot \nabla_t S}{D^{-1} + \int d\vec{r}\, \nabla_{\vec{r}} S \cdot \nabla_{\vec{r}} S}$$

with $\nabla_{\vec{r}} S$ and $\nabla_t S$ the space and time gradients of the spatiotemporal function $S(\vec{r}, t)$. This function is in effect the signal to noise ratio at the level of the photoreceptors, and is thus linearly related to the light intensities. In the full description the differentiation operations are implemented by biphasic filters, the details of which depend on the prior expectation of the values of several stimulus parameters. Qualitatively, we can see from the equation that if the SNR is high, the denominator is dominated by the integral term. At the same time the filters should become very localized. Together this means that at high SNR the computation approaches the gradient model. At low SNR, the denominator is dominated by D^{-1}, and the filters should widen up. In that case Eq. 3 takes the qualitative form of a correlation between two linearly filtered signals, integrated over the visual field, which is essentially Reichardt's correlator model.

If this type of flexibility is built in to the fly visual system, we should be able to adapt the fly's brain in different ways to regimes of different SNR and probe its properties. In terms of our optimal estimator this means that we adapt the fly to a certain set of statistical parameters, thereby changing its prior expectations. We then try to characterize the properties of the fly's movement computation for different priors. The model predicts for example that the gain and the dynamics of the response should adapt, and that we may expect a regime of correlator behavior and of pure velocity estimation. The experiments described below are an attempt to describe and interpret several aspects of adaptive behavior in H1.

3   Experimental methods

The experiments were performed on female wild type *Calliphora vicina*, caught outdoors. After immobilizing the wings with wax, the fly was put in a plastic tube, and its thorax and head were fixed with wax. Care was taken to leave the proboscis free so that the animal could be fed occasionally. The H1 neuron was recorded by an extracellular tungsten electrode reaching the lobula plate through a small hole cut in the back of the head.

In section 4.2 we analyze some previously published data. For the experiments described in other sections, patterns were generated using a Digital Signal Processor board (Ariel) based on a Motorola 56001 processor. Most consisted of frames of nominally 200 vertical lines, written at a frame rate of 500 Hz. Thus the patterns were essentially 1-dimensional, but extended in the vertical direction. In the experiments described in section 4.1 the pattern consisted of 380 dots, arranged in a 2-dimensional hexagonal pattern commensurate with the fly's sampling raster. Here the frame rate was 250 Hz. The patterns were displayed on a Tektronix 608 monitor (phosphor P31), at a radiance of 165 mW/(sr·cm^2). Taking spectral and optical characteristics of the photoreceptor lens-wave guide into account, we estimate a flux of effectively transduced photons of about $4.10^4 s^{-1}$ [24].

Prior to each set of experiments, the spatial sampling basis of the fly was measured by means of the reversed reaction. The distance of the fly to the screen was adjusted so that 4 lines on the screen corresponded to 1 horizontal interommatidial angle, which for the fly is about 1.35°. In most of the results presented below, this will be the unit in which we measure visual angle; it will be referred to as "omm". Consequently, most angular velocity values will be expressed in omm/s.

4   Experimental results

4.1   Computation of spatiotemporal correlations

Any form of movement computation based on an array of photoreceptor signals must compute relations between signals at different positions on the retina and at different delays. Here we design a stimulus pattern that makes this explicitly clear, and which allows us to map the space- and time dependency of the fly's movement sensitive neuron. The stimulus is a wide-field movement illusion which is generated by hidden correlations in an extended pattern. What is displayed on the CRT is an approximated version of the following pattern:

$$(4) \qquad I(\vec{r}, t) = m_1 \cdot I_0(\vec{r}, t) + m_2 \cdot I_0(\vec{r} - \Delta \vec{r}, t - \Delta t),$$

where $\vec{r}$ and t are two-dimensional position and time, $\Delta \vec{r}$ and Δt are spatial and temporal displacements. $I_0(\cdots, \cdots)$ is a white noise signal in space and time with spatiotemporal autocorrelation:

$$(5) \qquad \Phi_{I_0, I_0}(\vec{r}, t) = \delta(\vec{r}, t).$$

Then the autocorrelation of the pattern on the display approximates the following triplet of delta functions in space and time:

$$(6) \quad \Phi_{I,I}(\vec{r}, t) \;=\; (m_1^2 + m_2^2) \cdot \delta(\vec{r}, t)$$
$$+(m_1 \cdot m_2) \cdot (\delta(\vec{r} - \Delta\vec{r}, t - \Delta t) + \delta(\vec{r} + \Delta\vec{r}, t + \Delta t)).$$

The central peak describes a random flicker with strength $(m_1^2 + m_2^2)$, while the two satellite delta functions carry a movement signal, associated with an illusory velocity $\vec{v}_{ill} = \Delta\vec{r}/\Delta t$. Subjectively, this pattern gives a strong impression of wide-field movement, with flicker superimposed. Also the H1 neuron shows a clear direction-selective response to this stimulus. The motion signal, however, is only present as a statistical correlation at a specific offset in space and time. This demonstrates that the visual system must explicitly do something like computing a space-time correlation function on the retinal intensity signal. Figure 2 shows results of a measurement of H1's response to this stimulus, for different values of $\Delta\vec{r}$ and with $m_1 = m_2 = 0.5$ in Eq. 4. These data define a sensitivity map for the movement computation, and they demonstrate that H1 computes horizontal movement mainly by combining inputs from the nearest neighbors with oblique directions at $\pm 30°$ with the horizontal, substantially in agreement with previous reports [5].

This specific type of stimulus allows for more manipulations. We can, for example, change the sign of m_2 in Eq. 4. Then the locations of the delta functions in Eq. 6 remain unchanged, but the sign of the satellite peaks changes. This makes the perceived direction of motion reverse, and also H1 responds as if the motion goes in the opposite direction. Of course this stimulus is very unnatural, so it is not a priori clear what result we should expect, but the reversal of direction is predicted by a correlation model of movement detection.

Another thing we can do is manipulate m_1 and m_2 separately, keeping either the flicker term $(m_1^2 + m_2^2)$ or the motion-related term $m_1 \cdot m_2$ constant. Figure 3 compares these two cases, and it shows that the results of the two manipulations differ dramatically. If, keeping the motion term constant, the flicker term is set to a new level, H1 responds with a brisk over- or undershoot (Fig. 3a). The plateau levels of the response are virtually the same (3b). It thus seems that the fly's brain adapts to a change in the flicker stimulus in a few seconds, and that it strives to keep the motion related component constant. Changing $m_1 \cdot m_2$ at constant flicker power shows a different behavior. Here, H1's response steps almost instantaneously to a new value, and there is little adaptation. Thus, at constant flicker, the neuron seems to be measuring the motion related component instantaneously and without adaptation. These strategies seem to make sense for a neuron that is interested in motion and not in flicker. Note, however, that the neuron's output is not a pure representation of the $\vec{v}_{ill}$ as defined by the spatial and temporal offsets in the stimulus, but does depend on the product of the two modulation parameters.

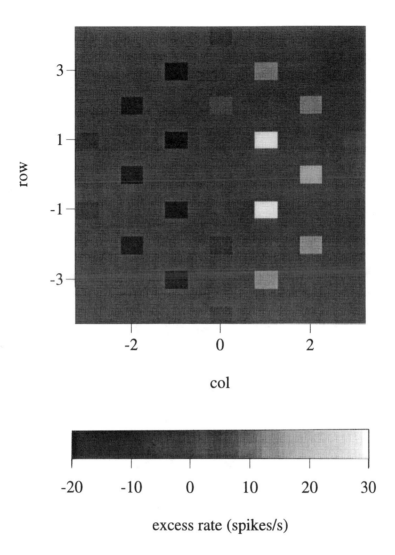

FIG. 2. *Response of H1 to an illusory wide-field motion stimulus. The plot shows the dependence of response on the location of spatial correlations as given by the row and column index (see text). Spatial coordinates are measured in units of the fly's spatial sampling raster. Gray-value indicates the firing rate of the nerve cell above the rate measured for position (0,0).*

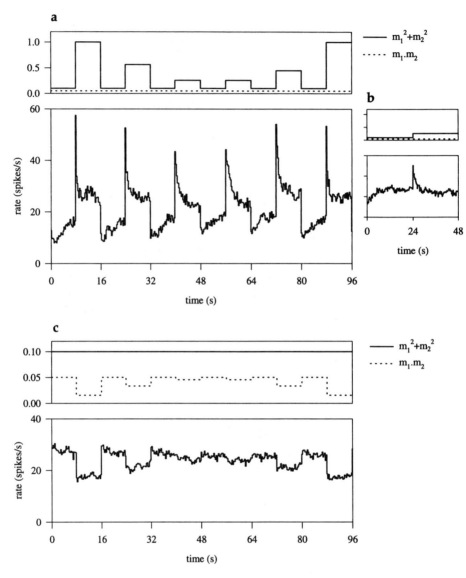

FIG. 3. *Response of H1 to changes in the intensity modulations m_1 and m_2 of an illusory wide-field motion stimulus, as defined in the text. Each subfigure consists of a stimulus trace on top, and a response post stimulus time histogram (psth) at the bottom. The stimuli were presented repeatedly, and the neuron's spike activity was averaged over all presentations.* **a:** *changes in the flicker contribution $(m_1^2 + m_2^2)$ induce strong transients.* **b:** *a similar stimulus as in* **a**, *but with only one transition every 24 s. This shows that the response reaches a plateau level that does not depend on the flicker strength.* **c:** *changes in the motion-related component $m_1 \cdot m_2$ are followed almost instantaneously and show no appreciable adaptation effects. Summarizing: the plateau response depends clearly on the motion related component, but hardly on the flicker component of the illusory motion stimulus*

4.2   Adaptation of response dynamics

It has been known for some time that the response of H1 adapts the dynamics of its response [32, 12, 25] over a wide range, with characteristic response decay times ranging from over 300 ms to about 10 ms. The time constant can be set by various dynamic parameters of the stimulus. In the case of stepwise movement, the time constant adapts to the time interval between steps, independent of step size or contrast [32]. Also, sinusoidal flicker of the full field [4], and random flicker of independent pixels (Fig. 4) influence the time constant. Further, in a situation where moving gratings are used as a stimulus, the time constant is set over a significant range by the velocity of the pattern, independent of its spatial wavelength or contrast [25]. Finally, the time constant is independent of the direction of movement, and is set locally in the visual field. Given the robustness and the magnitude of the effects, it would be highly surprising if this form of adaptation did not serve an important purpose. One possibility is that the effects seen in H1 are the result of adaptive low-pass filtering in retinotopic columns. The idea is that the statistical structure of the signals entering a photoreceptor is determined by the statistics of the visual scene, the optical properties of the photoreceptor, and the angular speed of the photoreceptor relative to the scene. Consequently, a measurement of pattern speed and salient contrast parameters provides the animal not only with data for direct use, but also gives it statistical information about the signals it could expect next. Specifically, if a pattern moves across the retina at angular velocity v, the power density spectrum of the optical signal transmitted by the photoreceptor optics is:

$$(7) \qquad S_{opt}(f) = \frac{C(f/v) \cdot M(f/v)}{v}$$

with $C(\kappa)$ the contrast power density of the pattern, $M(\kappa)$ the modulation power transfer function, κ the spatial frequency (in cycles/°), and f the induced temporal frequency in Hz. Thus a spatial frequency κ will be mapped to a temporal frequency $f = v \cdot \kappa$. Recently, power spectra of natural scenes, woods in this case, were measured [22, 23], and shown to have power-law behavior over at least three decades of spatial frequency. Converted to the one-dimensional case relevant here, $C(\kappa)$ is given as:

$$(8) \qquad C(\kappa) \propto \left(\frac{\kappa_0}{\kappa}\right)^{1-\eta}$$

with $\eta = 0.19$ and formally $\kappa_0 = 1$ cycle/° to make the term in brackets dimensionless. Further, $M(\kappa)$ is usually modeled as a Gaussian:

$$(9) \qquad M(\kappa) = \exp[-(2\pi\kappa)^2 \cdot \sigma_s^2]$$

with a spatial width $\sigma_s = 0.51°$. Next we must take into account the signal transfer properties and the noise power spectrum of the individual

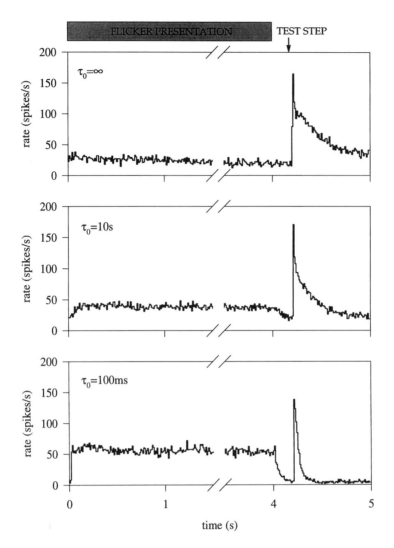

FIG. 4. *Adaptation of the dynamics of H1's response to the correlation time of a random stimulus. In the experiment the fly watched a random-bar pattern in which each bar was modulated independently with Gaussian noise for the first 4 seconds (see gray bar on top, labeled "flicker presentation"). Then the modulation was stopped, and at 4.2 seconds a small (0.5 omm, see sect. 3) movement step was presented (arrow). The decay time of the step response depends strongly on the correlation time, τ_0 of the Gaussian noise.*

photoreceptor. These were measured by intracellular recording, under the same illumination conditions that were used in the experiments on H1 [24]. For our purposes, signal transfer is described adequately by a linear contrast power transfer function $T(f)$, while the noise is Gaussian and given by the power density spectrum $N(f)$. Here we only need the ratio of these functions which is approximated by:

$$(10) \qquad N_{eff}(f) = \frac{N(f)}{T(f)} \approx 1.25 \cdot 10^{-4}[1 + (\frac{f}{f_c})^{2.7}]$$

with f_c about 18 Hz. This describes the equivalent noise power spectrum referred back to the stimulus. We now assume that the visual system measures the speed and contrast variance of the pattern, and that somewhere in the visual system a filter can be adapted to filter out those frequencies where the SNR of the photoreceptor input is too low. The cutoff frequency f_0 can be found by assuming the form of $C(\kappa)$ given above, scaling it with a prefactor to make the contrast variance equal to the measured value, and measuring the speed. Figure 5 presents the result of the computation of f_0, and compares it to data obtained from H1 [25]. The results are expressed as the measured quantity $\tau = 1/2\pi f_0$, which can be thought of as the integration time of a filter, adjusted to eliminate frequencies above f_0. Obviously the match between theory and experiment is far from perfect. But we must remember that the fly tries to solve a complicated problem, of which our model description can at best be a crude approximation. There are no free parameters in our calculation, and one could undoubtedly improve the fits of the computed curves to the measured values of τ. However, it is not our goal here to obtain good fits per se, and given the complexity of the system and the number of potential parameters this would not be very meaningful anyway.

Theory and experimental data do agree in several respects: First, for most of the range the orders of magnitude predicted for τ are within a factor of three from the measured values. Second, the theory predicts a weak dependence on contrast for low adaptation velocities, as found for H1. This is mainly due to the fact that at low velocities the optical signal is low-pass filtered with a very steep slope induced by the Gaussian modulation transfer function. Third, it predicts that the point of breakaway from the trend of decreasing τ with increasing velocity, does depend on contrast, which again is in line with the observations. Taken together, this indicates that the adaptive behavior of H1 is consistent with a mechanism that could serve an important purpose, namely suppressing high frequency components for which the SNR drops below a critical value. This is a very useful thing to do prior to combining signals in nonlinear interactions, because such interactions mix frequencies. For example, the low-frequency output of a second-order interaction results from the convolution of the two input spectra. Suppose that the inputs contain useful signals only at

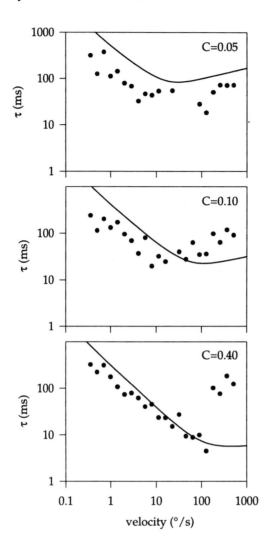

FIG. 5. *Dependence of adaptation time constant (τ) on the velocity of an adaptation stimulus. Dots: values of the measured characteristic decay time of H1's response to pattern steps (similar to those in Fig. 4), after preadapting the neuron with movement at a velocity given by the abscissa. Square-wave patterns (period 9.5°) were used with contrasts C as shown in the figure. Solid lines are time constants of optimal filters, computed as described in text.*

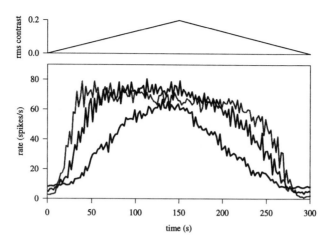

FIG. 6. *Response of H1 to movement in the preferred direction, at moderate speed (8 omm/s). During movement the contrast of the random bar pattern was ramped from 0 to 0.2 and back, as shown. Three levels of illumination were used: low (dark curve), middle (dark gray curve), and high (light gray curve). Illumination levels were spaced by factors of ten. At lower light levels the response rises less steeply, in other words the region of quadratic contrast dependence is larger. The maximum values of the response depend only weakly on illumination level.*

low frequencies and that broad band noise is added. Then, even if the low frequency SNR of the inputs to the computation is high, the output of the computation may be completely dominated by the noise, because in the interaction the noise-noise cross product is integrated over the full bandwidth. This argument is quite general in the sense that the statistics of photon arrival induces broad band noise in the photoreceptors so that prefiltering signals prior to nonlinearities is probably important in practice. Further, prefiltering should be adaptive if the computations are to span a reasonable dynamic range.

4.3   Adaptation to light intensity

In this experiment the fly watched a pattern moving in the preferred direction of H1, at a speed of 8 omm/s. The pattern consisted of vertical lines with intensities set independently from the others according to a Gaussian distribution. The contrast was slowly (period 300 s) ramped up and down from zero up to an rms value of 0.5. However, because the line width was set at one quarter of the interommatidial angle, the lines were substantially blurred by the photoreceptor optics, resulting in an estimated maximum rms contrast value of 0.2. The experiment was done for three values of the light intensity, by having the fly look at the screen either directly, or through

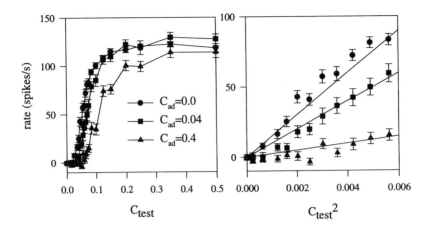

FIG. 7. *Dependence of H1's movement response on test contrast, when adapted to different adaptation contrasts. The data in the right figure are for the low contrast regime only, and the abscissa is quadratic. The fact that straight lines on this plot fit the data well means that for this test contrast range, H1 responds like a correlator. The gain of the correlator is seen to depend on the adaptation contrast.*

a filter with either 10% or 1% transmission. Figure 6 shows the result of this experiment for the three light levels. Without filter the response of H1 increases steeply as contrast increases and reaches a plateau value at relatively low contrast values. A noteworthy feature of the curve is also that it is not symmetric: the response to the downward contrast flank is different from that to the upward one. As the stimulus period was 300 seconds, this means that long-term adaptation effects play a role in shaping the response. For lower light intensities, it can be seen that the range over which the response depends more or less quadratically on contrast increases with decreasing light levels. This is expected from the simple picture: at lower light levels, the relative SNR decreases, thus widening the contrast range over which correlation operations rather than gradient schemes are optimal. In the experiment presented here, the range should scale to first approximation inversely with intensity, which is roughly correct. Although the response at the lowest light level increases slower than at the higher levels, its value at maximum contrast is not that different from the other cases. This is an interesting phenomenon, and it could point to a mechanism in which the effect of contrast on H1's response is suppressed, as soon as the SNR becomes high enough. The following experiment was designed to test this more explicitly.

4.4   Adaptation to contrast

A more detailed way of looking at contrast dependence is to probe adaptation to contrast. As an adaptation stimulus, in this experiment the fly saw a Gaussian random pattern move at constant velocity (8 omm/s) in the null direction of the neuron. Adaptation movement in the preferred direction gave qualitatively the same results, although there were differences in detail. Most likely, these resulted from tonic high firing rate induced by such an adaptation stimulus. After 3 seconds of adaptation movement the velocity changed sign, and the contrast changed to a test contrast value. This test phase lasted for 1 second, whereupon the adaptation stimulus resumed. The estimated values of adaptation contrast at the photoreceptor level in this experiment were: 0.0, 0.01, 0.02, 0.03, 0.06, and 0.2. We can now ask for the dependence of H1's movement response on the test contrast, given a certain value of the adaptation contrast. In order to avoid as far as possible the effect of transients induced by the contrast switch from adaptation to test, the movement response was computed over the last 500 ms of the presentation of the test stimulus. The results are shown in Fig. 7 at two test contrast resolutions. The top figure shows again that the test response reaches a plateau as a function of test contrast, and the plateau values do not depend very much on adaptation contrast. On the other hand, the contrast gain of the test response depends strongly on the adaptation contrast in the region of low test contrasts, as can be seen from the bottom figure. This graph also shows that in the low contrast region, H1 shows typical correlator-like behavior, in that the movement response is a quadratic function of contrast. In this regime the gain of the correlator is very sensitive to the adaptation contrast. Here, the gain varies from $2.5 \cdot 10^4 - 0.3 \cdot 10^4$ spikes s^{-1} (rms contrast)$^{-2}$, with adaptation contrast increasing from 0.0 to 0.2.

4.5   Influence of contrast and velocity

The time sequence of the experiment was slightly more complicated. In order to keep the neuron in a reasonably steady state of adaptation we presented null-direction movement at a constant velocity for periods of 3 seconds, interleaved with preferred direction movement during 1 second. Meanwhile the contrast of the pattern changed in triangular fashion, with a period of 100 seconds. This means that we probed the response to preferred direction movement 25 times each period. The result, expressed as the averaged firing rate during each preferred-direction stimulation as a function of both contrast and velocity, is shown in Fig. 8. At low contrast, as shown in the top figure, the output of H1 is ambiguous in the sense that it depends both on contrast and velocity. The response starts to show a plateau as a function of contrast for contrast values above 0.2. However, even in this plateau region, the response still depends strongly on velocity over a wide dynamic range. So it seems that at higher contrasts, H1 has normalized contrast away, and

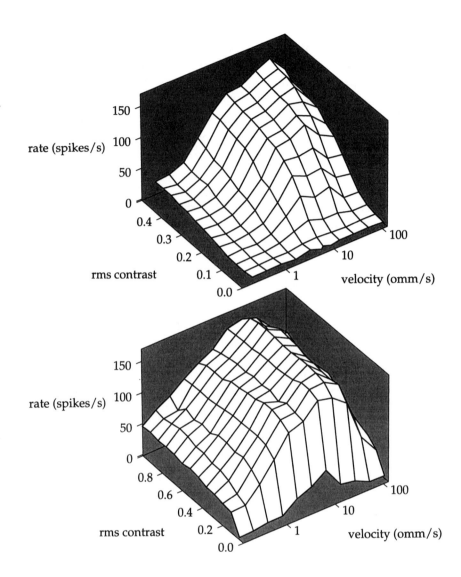

FIG. 8. *Firing rate of H1 as a function of both contrast and velocity. Velocity was presented alternatingly in null direction (3 s, v=8 omm/s, and preferred direction (1 s, v as given by axis). Rate in both figures is averaged over the last 500 ms of motion in the preferred direction. Top figure shows an experiment with finer resolution of contrasts. At low contrast it shows a quadratic contrast dependence. Bottom figure shows results over a wider contrast range and demonstrates that the response hardly depends on contrasts for contrasts higher than about 0.2. This is not due to saturation in the neuron itself, as the response clearly depends strongly on velocity, even at the higher contrasts.*

is sensitive to velocity only. This is in line with the behavior predicted by Eq. 3. We should be careful interpreting these results, as there are more parameters that influence H1's response, such as the spatial structure of the stimulus.

5   Conclusion

Probably the most important conclusion we can draw from our results, is that the visual system of the fly may be very adaptive in its computations. Furthermore, we tentatively understand some of the effects we see in terms of optimal processing of noisy photoreceptor signals.

Another important lesson is that we can manipulate experimental conditions such that H1 shows distinct features of either a correlator, or a pure velocity sensor. This may mean that proponents of the correlator scheme, and those in favor of gradient models [6] really look at two sides of the same coin, namely the adaptive movement sensor, described by Eq. 3.

Acknowledgments

We would like to thank Al Schweitzer for his wonderful technical support and Hans van Hateren for his help with the photoreceptor measurements. M.P was supported in part by a NSERC '67 Fellowship.

References

[1] H. B. Barlow and W. R. Levick, *Three factors limiting the reliable detection of light by retinal ganglion cells of the cat* J. Physiol., 200 (1969), pp. 1-24.

[2] W. Bialek, F. Rieke, R. R. de Ruyter van Steveninck and D. Warland, D. *Reading a neural code*, Science, 252 (1991), pp. 854-1857.

[3] W. Bialek, M. Potters, D. Ruderman, and R. R. de Ruyter van Steveninck *Visual computation: A fly's eye view* In Cognitive Processing for Vision and Voice, Proceedings of the Fourth NEC Symposium, ed. T. Ishiguro, pp. 7-26. SIAM Philadelphia, 1993.

[4] A. Borst and M. Egelhaaf 1987 *Temporal modulation of luminance adapts time constant of fly movement detectors* Biol. Cybern., 56 (1987), pp. 209-215.

[5] E. Buchner *Elementary movement detectors in an insect visual system*, Biol. Cybern., 24 (1976), pp. 85-101.

[6] E. Buchner *Behavioural analysis of spatial vision in insects*, in Photoreception and vision in invertebrates M.A. Ali ed., pp. 561-622. Plenum Press New York, NY, 1984.

[7] K. Hausen *Motion sensitive interneurons in the optomotor system of the fly. I. The horizontal cells: Structure and signals* Biol. Cybern., 45 (1982), pp. 143-156.

[8] K. Hausen *Motion sensitive interneurons in the optomotor system of the fly. II. The horizontal cells: Receptive field organization and response characteristics*

Biol. Cybern., 46 (1982), pp. 67-79.

[9] K. Hausen and C. Wehrhahn *Microsurgical lesion of horizontal cells changes optomotor yaw responses in the blowfly* Calliphora erytrocephala Proc. R. Soc. Lond., B 219 (1983), pp. 211-216.

[10] S. Hecht, S. Shlaer and M. H. Pirenne *Energy, quanta, and vision*, J. Gen. Physiol., 25 (1942), pp. 819-840.

[11] J.O. Limb, and J.A. Murphy 1975 *Estimating the velocity of moving objects in television signals*, Comp.Graph.Image.Proc., 4 (1975), pp. 311-327.

[12] T. Maddess and S. B. Laughlin *Adaptation of the motion sensitive neuron H1 is generated locally and governed by contrast frequency*, Proc. R. Soc. Lond., B 225 (1985), pp. 251-275.

[13] K. Nakayama *Biological image motion processing: a review*, Vision Res., 25 (1985), pp. 625-660.

[14] R. Pierantoni *A look into the cock-pit of the fly. The architecture of the lobula plate*, Cell Tissue Res., 171 (1976), pp. 101-122.

[15] T. Poggio and W. Reichardt *Visual control of orientation behaviour in the fly, Part II. Towards the underlying neural interactions*, Q. Rev.Biophys. 9, (1976), pp. 377-438.

[16] M. Potters *Toward a predictive theory of neural computation: motion estimation in the fly's visual system*, thesis, University of Princeton, Princeton NJ, 1994.

[17] M. Potters and W. Bialek *Statistical Mechanics and Visual Signal Processing*, J. Phys. I France, 4 (1994), pp. 1755-1775.

[18] W. Reichardt *Autokorrelations Auswertung als Funktionsprinzip des Zentralnervensystems*, Z. Naturf., 12b (1957), pp. 448-457.

[19] W. Reichardt 1961 *Autocorrelation, a principle for the evaluation of sensory information by the central nervous system*, in Sensory communication, ed. W.A. Rosenblith, pp. 303-317. MIT Press, Cambridge MA 1961.

[20] W. Reichardt and T. Poggio *Visual control of orientation behaviour in the fly, Part I. A quantitative analysis*, Q. Rev.Biophys. 9, (1976), pp. 311-375.

[21] A. Rose *The sensitivity performance of the human eye on an absolute scale*, J. Opt. Soc. Am., 38 (1948), pp. 196-208.

[22] D.L. Ruderman *Natural ensembles and sensory signal processing*, thesis, University of California, Berkeley, 1993.

[23] D.L. Ruderman and W. Bialek, *Statistics of natural images: Scaling in the woods*, Phys. Rev. Lett., 73 (1994), pp. 814-817.

[24] R. R. de Ruyter van Steveninck *Real-time performance of a movement-sensitive neuron in the blowfly visual system*, thesis, Rijksuniversiteit Groningen, The Netherlands, 1986.

[25] R. R. de Ruyter van Steveninck, W.H. Zaagman and H.A.K. Mastebroek, 1986 *Adaptation of transient responses of a movement-sensitive neuron in the visual system of the blowfly* Calliphora erythrocephala, Biol. Cybern., 54 (1986), 223-236.

[26] R. R. de Ruyter van Steveninck and W. Bialek *Statistical reliability of a blowfly movement-sensitive neuron*, in Advances in Neural Information Processing Systems Moody, J.E., Hanson, S.J., Lippmann, R.P. eds., pp. 27-34. Morgan Kaufmann, San Mateo, California 1992.

[27] R. R. de Ruyter van Steveninck and W. Bialek, *Reliability and Statistical Efficiency of a Blowfly Movement-Sensitive Neuron*, Phil Trans. R. Soc. Lond. B, in press.

[28] R. R. de Ruyter van Steveninck and S.B. Laughlin, in prep.

[29] G. L. Savage and M.S. Banks *Scotopic visual efficiency: Constraints by optics, receptor properties and rod pooling*, Vision Res., 32-4 (1992), pp. 645-656.

[30] Hl. de Vries 1943 *The quantum character of light and its bearing upon threshold of vision, the differential sensitivity and visual acuity of the eye*, Physica, 10 (1943), pp. 553-564.

[31] H.A. van der Velden 1944 *Over het aantal lichtquanta dat nodig is voor een lichtprikkel bij het menselijk oog*, Physica, 11 (1944), pp. 179-189.

[32] W. H. Zaagman, H. A. K. Mastebroek and R. R. de Ruyter van Steveninck *Adaptive strategies in fly vision: On their image processing qualities*, IEEE Trans. Man Syst. Cybern., SMC13 (1983), pp. 900-906.

Chapter 3
Activity-Dependent Conductances
in Model and Biological Neurons

L.F. Abbott, G. Turrigiano, G. LeMasson and E. Marder[1]

1. Introduction

It is widely believed that activity-dependent plasticity in neuronal circuits is the basic phenomenon underlying learning and memory (Morris et al., 1986; Byrne and Berry, 1989; Gluck and Rumelhart, 1990; Baudry and Davis, 1991; Hawkins, Kandel and Siegelbaum, 1993). In addition, neural modifications guided by activity are thought to play a crucial role in the development of neural networks (Shatz, 1990; Miller, 1990). Research on the role of activity-dependent plasticity in learning, memory and development has focused primarily on modifications of synaptic efficacy. Connectionist neural networks have revealed some of the computational functions that can be achieved by networks developed using various learning rules that modify synaptic strengths (Gluck and Rumelhart, 1990; Churchland and Sejnowski, 1992). At the same time, enormous experimental effort has been devoted to studying long-term potentiation and depression of synapses (Byrne and Berry 1989; Malenka and Nicoll, 1993; Artola and Singer, 1993) and exploring how these processes might modify behavior (Morris et al., 1986; Abbott and Blum, 1994). While activity-dependent synaptic changes are of great importance to learning, memory and development, they are not the only form of activity-dependent plasticity relevant to network function. The intrinsic characteristics of individual neurons can also be modified by activity (Alkon, 1984; Franklin, Fickbohm and Willard, 1992; Turrigiano, Abbott and Marder, 1994). The behavior of a neural network depends both on synaptic connections and on the intrinsic electrical characteristics of individual network neurons. Along with synaptic plasticity, activity-dependent modification of intrinsic properties has important implications for neural network behavior (Levy, Colbert and Desmond, 1990; LeMasson, Marder and Abbott, 1993; Abbott and LeMasson, 1993; Siegel, Marder and Abbott,

[1]Center for Complex Systems and Biology Department, Brandeis University, Waltham, MA 02254.

1994) .

Individual neurons are complex dynamic systems that exhibit a wide range of endogenous behaviors including tonic (periodic) spiking, periodic firing in bursts and bistability between silent and firing states, even in the absence of synaptic input (Llinás, 1988; Harris-Warrick and Marder, 1991). A dozen or more different types of ion channels contribute to the membrane conductance of a typical neuron (Llinás, 1988; McCormick, 1990; Hille, 1992). Neuronal electrical characteristics depend on the number of channels of each type active within the plasma membrane and on how these channels are distributed over the surface of the cell. Modeling studies indicate that even small changes in the numbers, conductances or distributions of ion channels can have a dramatic effect on neuronal behavior.

Living cells exist in a state of dynamic equilibrium in which macroscopic properties are maintained despite continual molecular turnover. In the case of neurons, new ion channels are continually being synthesized, transported to various parts of the cell and inserted into the membrane while old channels are removed and disassembled. In light of this continual channel turnover, the robust stability of biological neurons is rather surprising. Furthermore, neurons must adjust to their own growth and to possible changes in the extracellular environment over the course of their lifetimes. A complex array of biochemical processes controls the number and distribution of ion channels by constructing and transporting channels, modulating their properties and inserting them into and removing them from the plasma membrane. Many of these processes are affected by electrical activity. For example, electrical activity can induce gene expression (Sheng and Greenberg, 1990; Morgan and Curran, 1991; Hemmick et al., 1992; Armstrong and Montminy, 1993) and lead to activity-dependent modulation of active ion channels (Kaczmarek and Levitan, 1987).

The molecular mechanisms responsible for ion channel synthesis, modulation and degradation are typically ignored in neuron models because it is generally assumed that these processes maintain the density of ion channels over the surface of the cell membrane at approximately constant levels. As a result, channel densities are treated as fixed parameters in these models. We would like to challenge this viewpoint and suggest instead that the molecular biology of the neuron might be geared to maintaining constant average activity rather than constant channel densities. It is difficult to see how a neuron could actually monitor the density of its ion channels other than through the effect of these channels on electrical activity. Furthermore, it seems more likely that the molecular processes controlling channel density would have evolved to maintain the neuronal activity needed for a specific task rather than to maintain the specific numbers of channels active in the membrane. We have constructed and studied models that incorporate this alternate conception of the role of the molecular machinery of the cell (LeMasson, Marder and Abbott, 1993; Abbott and LeMasson, 1993; Siegel, Marder and Abbott, 1994). In addition, we have conducted a series of experiments that strongly support this alternate viewpoint (Turrigiano, Abbott and Marder, 1994). Both the modeling and experimental studies have important implications concerning the role of activity-dependent plasticity in network function.

2. The Model

Modeling the mechanism by which ion channels are constructed, transported, inserted into the cell membrane, modulated and finally removed from the membrane would be an enormously complicated undertaking. Fortunately, we can learn about the role of these processes and in particular the effect of their dependence on activity without constructing a detailed mechanistic model. Two features help to simplify the construction of such models. First, the essential element we need in order to understand the impact of activity-dependent intrinsic properties is the feedback mechanism that links a neuron's electrical characteristics to its activity. If we can uncover the basic rules by which activity modulates these characteristics, we can study their impact without having to build detailed mechanistic models. A similar approach is used to study synaptic plasticity where the implications of a synaptic learning rule can be studied without a precise knowledge of the molecular mechanisms of synaptic modification. Second, channel synthesis, insertion, modulation and removal are much slower than the usual voltage- and ligand-dependent processes that open and close channels. Thus, activity-dependent regulation of conductances introduces a new, slower dynamic time scale into neuronal modeling. Because activity-dependent changes are so much slower than the processes responsible for action potentials, bursting and other similar phenomena, the dynamics splits into two widely different temporal scales and this simplifies the analysis of activity-dependent models (Abbott and LeMasson, 1993).

The basic idea of activity-dependent conductances is that the electrical activity of a neuron plays a feedback role in regulating its currents. It is difficult to imagine how a neuron could ever develop and maintain the membrane currents it needs to function properly without such a feedback loop. The feedback element giving rise to activity-dependent conductances should be sensitive to the electrical activity of the neuron and must be capable of regulating numerous biochemical processes. Intracellular calcium is a prime candidate for such an element. Since calcium enters the neuron through voltage-dependent channels, the average level of intracellular calcium is highly correlated with the level of electrical activity of the neuron (Ross 1989; LeMasson, Marder and Abbott, 1993). Calcium works much better than other ions for this purpose because intracellular calcium concentrations are very low, giving it the required sensitivity. Calcium is also a ubiquitous regulator of biochemical pathways and it appears to play a role in many processes affecting membrane conductances. Changes in the intracellular calcium concentration are associated with both modifications of channel properties (Chad and Eckert, 1986; Gruol, Deal and Yool, 1992; Kaczmarek and Levitan, 1987) and long-term changes in gene expression (Murphy, Worley and Baraban, 1991). The models we have constructed to study activity-dependent conductances (LeMasson, Marder and Abbott, 1993; Abbott and LeMasson, 1993; Siegel, Marder and Abbott, 1994) use intracellular calcium as the feedback element linking neuronal characteristics to electrical activity. In addition, we have found experimental evidence that calcium plays a crucial role in activity-dependent changes of intrinsic neuronal characteristics in biological neurons (Turrigiano, Abbott and Marder, 1994).

In a single-compartment, conductance-based neuron models, the membrane potential V of a neuron is governed by the equation (for reviews see Koch and Segev, 1989; Abbott, 1994)

$$C\frac{dV}{dt} = -\sum_i I_i \tag{2.1}$$

where C is the membrane capacitance per unit area and the sum on the right side is the total membrane current per unit area. The individual terms I_i refer to the different types of membrane currents present in the neuron. Each individual current I_i is written in the form first developed by Hodgkin and

Huxley (1952)

$$I_i = \overline{g}_i m_i^{p_i} h_i^{q_i} (V - E_i) \qquad (2.2)$$

where E_i is the equilibrium potential for current i, p_i and q_i are integers and $\overline{g}_i$ is the maximal conductance for the current. The dynamic variables m_i and h_i are determined by first-order rate equations (Hodgkin and Huxley, 1952). The maximal conductance $\overline{g}_i$ is equal to the single-channel open conductance of the ion channels responsible for current i times the density of these channels in the membrane. Any processes that add, move or remove ion channels from the membrane or that modify the open conductance of a channel will change the values of the maximal conductances. Thus, activity-dependent modification of channel conductances, numbers and/or distributions can be modeled by allowing the maximal conductances $\overline{g}_i$ to vary with activity. Activity-dependent modification of channel kinetics can be introduced by allowing the voltage-dependent rate constants in these models to be modified by the activity-dependent feedback element intracellular calcium. However, we have only studied models with activity-dependent maximal conductances thus far.

In conductance-based neuron models since the time of Hodgkin and Huxley (1952), the maximal conductances $\overline{g}_i$ have been considered to be fixed parameters. This is in agreement with the viewpoint that a neuron maintains its ion channel densities at fixed values throughout its lifetime. Since we are challenging this viewpoint by suggesting that it is the average activity of the cell rather than the maximal conductances that are held constant, the $\overline{g}_i$ are dynamic variables in our neuron models (LeMasson, Marder and Abbott, 1993; Abbott and LeMasson, 1993; Siegel, Marder and Abbott, 1994). Because intracellular calcium is used as a feedback element in these models, the steady-state values of the maximal conductances $\overline{g}_i$ depend on the intracellular calcium concentration. We assume that the maximal conductances approach calcium-dependent steady-state values exponentially with a large time constant, on the order of many minutes or even hours. The long time of exponential approach reflects the fact that the processes like channel synthesis or degradation that are responsible for changing neuronal conductances are slow.

How do the steady-state values of the maximal conductances depend on the intracellular calcium concentration? Clearly, conductances cannot go below zero and, in addition, we assume that they cannot rise above some maximum value. This suggests that we use sigmoidal functions to model the dependence of the steady-state maximal conductances on the intracellular calcium concentration. For simplicity, we choose the sigmoidal functions for all the different conductances to have the general same form. Thus we write

$$\tau \frac{d\bar{g}_i}{dt} = \frac{G_i}{1 + \exp\left(\pm([Ca^{2+}] - C_T)/\Delta\right)} - \bar{g}_i .$$ (2.3)

Here $[Ca^{2+}]$ is the intracellular calcium concentration, τ is the large time constant that reflects the slow dynamics of the activity-dependent processes and C_T and Δ are parameters controlling the shape of the sigmoidal function. As mentioned above, a key element in the model is that changes of the $\bar{g}_i$ are slow, that is, τ is larger than any of the time constants characterizing other dynamic processes in the model. The behavior of these models is not very sensitive to the exact value of Δ. The more important role of the parameter C_T will be discussed shortly. The parameters G_i in (2.3) are the maximum possible values of the maximal conductances mentioned above. While the model is not overly sensitive to their precise values, their ratios can affect the behavior exhibited.

Remaining to be determined in equation (2.3) is the plus/minus sign in the exponential. We use the plus sign in this equation for inward currents and the minus sign for outward currents. The reasons for this particular choice is stability. Excessive activity tends to increase the calcium concentration in a neuron. If we use the plus sign for inward currents and minus sign for outward currents in equation (2.3), an increase in $[Ca^{2+}]$ has the effect of decreasing the strength of inward currents and increasing the strength of outward currents. Both of these changes tend to reduce the activity of the neuron thereby compensating for the excessive activity. A decrease in the activity of the neuron will have the opposite effect, decreasing $[Ca^{2+}]$ and thereby decreasing outward and increasing inward currents. This has the stabilizing affect of increasing activity. Thus our choice of plus and minus signs assures that calcium will provide a negative, stabilizing feedback loop.

Since the intracellular calcium concentration plays such an important role, we must model it as well. Calcium enters the cell through voltage-dependent membrane currents that we will call collectively I_{Ca}, diffuses through the cell and is removed by a buffering mechanism that we model as exponential decay. Thus,

$$\frac{d[Ca^{2+}]}{dt} = -AI_{Ca} - B[Ca^{2+}] \qquad (2.4)$$

Here B is the calcium uptake rate and the factor A converts from Coulombs of current to moles/liter of calcium concentration. Because calcium enters through the surface of the cell while concentration refers to the volume inside the cell, A is proportional to the surface-to-volume ratio of the neuron.

In conventional neuron models, the maximal conductances $\overline{g}_i$ are parameters that can be varied until the model produces a pattern of activity that matches the biological neuron being studied. In our models, the maximal conductances are dynamic variables and they take whatever values equation (2.3) assigns to them. What then determines the pattern of activity that the model neuron exhibits? Although other parameters of the models, the G_i in particular, play a role, the parameter that primarily determines the output of the model neuron is C_T appearing in equation (2.3). Equation (2.3) is really a self-consistency condition. The maximal conductances $\overline{g}_i$ determine the type of electrical activity that the neuron will produce through equations (2.1) and (2.2). This activity affects the level of intracellular calcium through equation (2.4). Finally, the calcium level feeds back to modify the maximal conductances through equation (2.3). The entire system will come to equilibrium when the maximal conductances take steady-state values that produce a level of activity leading to an average intracellular calcium concentration consistent with these conductances. This equilibrium point is largely determined by the value of C_T. Thus, the output of a model neuron, even with many different conductances, can be controlled by adjusting the single parameter C_T.

3. Model Results

Model neurons with dynamic maximal conductances display a number of interesting features. To illustrate these we will consider first a particularly simple version based on the Morris-Lecar (1981) model. This model has voltage-dependent calcium and potassium currents (for a review see Rinzel and Ermentrout, 1989). The active component of the membrane current is

$$I = \overline{g}_{Ca}M(V)(V - E_{Ca}) + \overline{g}_K n(V - E_K) \qquad (3.1)$$

where M(V) is a sigmoidal function of V and n is a dynamic variable determined by a first-order equation with voltage-dependent parameters. In the original, unregulated form of the model, the maximal conductances $\overline{g}_{Ca}$ and $\overline{g}_K$ are constants. In the activity/calcium regulated version, they are allowed to vary slowly as a function of the intracellular calcium concentration as in equation (2.3) with different values of the parameter G_{Ca} and G_K, but the same values of τ, C_T and Δ. The plus sign in equation (2.3) is used for $\overline{g}_{Ca}$ and the minus sign for $\overline{g}_K$.

The activity/calcium regulated models we have studied are self-assembling. In the two-conductance model of equation (3.1), the firing frequency depends on the value of the parameter C_T and a wide variety of frequencies can be achieved by adjusting this parameter. Once C_T is fixed, the model will automatically adjust its conductances to fire at the given frequency. Self-assembly is evident because the conductances required to achieve this frequency of firing arise spontaneously in the model from virtually any initial set of conductances. This is seen in figure 1 where four different starting configurations are shown all ultimately evolving to the same set of steady-state conductances which produce the same firing frequency.

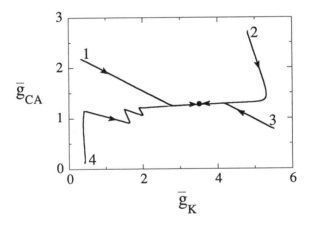

Figure 1: Self-assembly of conductances in a two-conductance model. The point marked by the dot denotes the steady-state calcium and potassium maximal conductances of the model. These are established from four different starting points (denoted by numbers) along paths depicted by lines with arrows. (Adapted from Abbott and LeMasson, 1993).

Model neurons with activity/calcium-dependent regulation of conductances are much more stable than their unregulated counterparts. Figure 2 contrasts the behavior of the regulated and unregulated models for different values of the potassium and calcium equilibrium potentials E_K and E_{Ca}. This simulates changes in the extracellular concentrations of these ions. The firing frequency of the unregulated model is extremely sensitive to these values. For the regulated model, the adjustment of maximal conductances maintains approximately the same firing frequency over a wide range of E_K and E_{Ca}. This occurs because the regulatory mechanism adjusts the maximal conductances of the calcium and potassium currents whenever the internal calcium concentration changes. Because the intracellular calcium concentration is tightly correlated with the activity of the neuron, maintaining a constant $[Ca^{2+}]$ automatically stabilizes the firing frequency of the neuron.

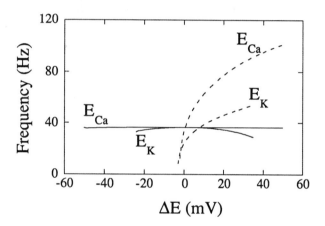

Figure 2: The effect of changing the reversal potentials for potassium and calcium on the activity of the two-conductance model neuron. The horizontal axis is the amount of the shift in either E_{Ca} or E_K while the vertical axis shows the resulting firing frequency. The original unregulated model is highly sensitive to these shifts as shown by the dashed curves. The model with activity-dependent conductances fires at almost the same frequency over the entire range as shown by the solid lines. (Adapted from Abbott and LeMasson, 1993).

Figure 3 shows the same stability property in a much more complex model, an activity/calcium regulated and somewhat modified version of a model of the LP neuron of the crustacean stomatogastric ganglion (Buchholtz et al., 1992). The LP (Lateral Pyloric) is a motor neuron of the stomatogastric ganglion that participates in a roughly 1 Hz rhythm responsible for food filtering motions in the pyloric region of the foregut of the lobster and crab. The model LP neuron has seven active conductances and is capable of firing action potentials either tonically or in periodic bursts. Figure 3 shows a plot of voltage versus time for this model neuron. The parameter C_T was adjusted to make the neuron fire in periodic bursts as shown by the activity at the start of the top trace. At the time indicated, we simulate an increase in the amount of extracellular potassium by changing the potassium reversal potential E_K. This causes the neuron to go into a fast, tonic firing mode. Due to the increased activity, the intracellular calcium concentration increases and, through equation (2.3), the maximal conductances $\overline{g}_i$ are modified. The result of this modification is a return to a bursting mode of activity as seen in the bottom trace. Thus, the model neuron has recovered from an environmental change by regulating its conductances to preserve its pattern of electrical activity. The set of maximal conductances that produces

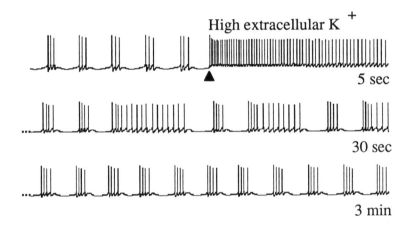

Figure 3: The effect of changing the reversal potential for potassium on the activity of the LP model neuron. Initially the model is in a bursting state. The simulated rise in extracellular potassium at the time marked by the triangle causes the activity to switch to tonic firing. After a readjustment period, bursting is restored. (Adapted from LeMasson, Marder and Abbott, 1993.)

the activity in the bottom trace is completely different than those present initially at the beginning of the top trace. The new parameter values were found automatically on the basis of feedback from activity through the intracellular calcium concentration. Note that to speed up these simulations, the dynamics of the conductance regulation in all the figures is faster than we expect it to be in real neurons.

Figure 4 shows that the same regulatory scheme that produces stability to perturbations also induces activity-dependent intrinsic properties. Once again, the model neuron is initially a burster as seen at the beginning of the top trace. At the times indicated by bars, pulses of external current are injected, increasing the activity of the neuron. This increased activity raises the intracellular calcium concentration thereby changing the maximal conductances $\overline{g}_i$. We show this by stopping the pulses in the bottom trace. After the stimulation, the model neuron has different intrinsic properties, it no longer fires spontaneously in bursts but is silent instead.

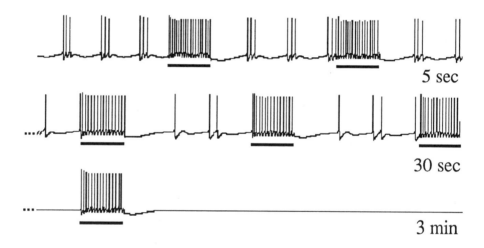

Figure 4: The effect of stimulation on the intrinsic properties of the LP model neuron. Periodic stimulation of the model, indicated by the bars, changed its intrinsic behavior from bursting (before stimulation) to silent (after stimulation). (Adapted from LeMasson, Marder and Abbott, 1993.)

Activity/calcium-dependent regulation will change membrane conductances whenever the activity of a neuron is modified for a long enough period of time to produce a sustained change in the level of intracellular calcium. This modification could be caused by changes in the extracellular environment as in figures 2 and 3 or by inputs as in figure 4. The adjustments will always be in the direction of restoring or maintaining the original level of activity and holding the intracellular calcium concentration relatively constant. Short-lasting changes of activity like brief bursts of action potentials will have little effect on conductances due to the slow response of the variables $\overline{g}_i$.

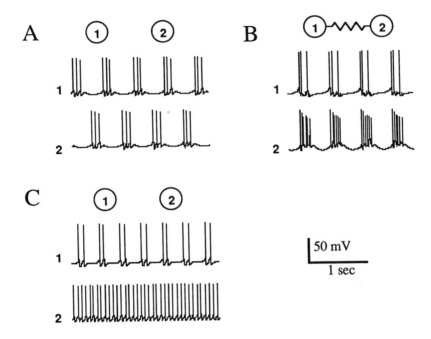

Figure 5: Spontaneous differentiation of two identical model neurons in a two-cell network. A) Two identical model neurons fire in identical bursts when they are uncoupled. B) After coupling through an electrical synapse, the activity of the two neurons is no longer identical. C) Removing the coupling and quickly examining the behavior of the neurons reveals that they have spontaneously differentiated with one becoming an intrinsic burster and the other tonically firing. (Adapted from Abbott and LeMasson, 1993.)

The fact that activity can shift the intrinsic electrical characteristics of neurons has important implications for networks. We show this in a simple two-cell network in figure 5. Two identical model LP neurons are symmetrically coupled through an electrical synapse. We begin, in figure 5A, with two bursting model neurons that are identical and uncoupled. In figure 5B, we show what happens after they are coupled electrically and allowed to interact for an extended period of time. Even though the two neurons are described by identical underlying models and the coupling is completely symmetric, their activity in the network is not identical. This difference is caused by the fact that the interaction between the two neurons has modified their intrinsic properties through the activity-dependent mechanism present in the model. To see what is going on, we eliminate the electrical coupling and show in figure 5C the behavior of the two neurons immediately after the coupling is removed. Clearly neuron 1 has retained a bursting pattern of activity, but neuron 2 has changed from a bursting to a tonically firing cell. The coupling between the two neurons has shifted their intrinsic properties so that the two initially bursting neurons have spontaneously differentiated to form a circuit in which one acts as a pacemaker and the other as a follower.

The models discussed up to now have all been single compartment models with uniform distributions of conductances. However, real neurons have complex spatial structures and their ion channels are not spread uniformly over the surface of their membranes but rather have a specific spatial distribution. Since the models described here control channel density as reflected by the maximal conductance parameters, it is interesting to investigate whether they can account for the spatial structure of channel distributions. This can be done by applying the rule (2.3) governing maximal conductance values locally, compartment-by-compartment in a multi-compartment neuron model using the calcium concentration within each compartment as the local feedback signal. In a spatially structured model neuron, the calcium concentration is affected both by influx through voltage-dependent channels and by the geometry of the cell because of surface-to-volume effects and diffusion. Thus, the distribution of conductances in such models will depend on the activity of the neuron, on its morphology and on the spatial pattern of synaptic input that it receives.

We have studied such models in collaboration with M. Siegel (Siegel, Marder and Abbott, 1994). We find that local calcium regulation of channel density through equation (2.3) in multi-compartmental models can produce a realistic spatial distribution of channels. In a complex model of a hippocampal CA1 pyramidal neuron, a passive dendritic tree and an active axon with an action-potential initiation region at and near the soma arose spontaneously from an initial state in which all conductances were zero (for a different approach to this problem see Bell, 1992). Thus, the multi-compartment model revealed the same self-assembly properties as the one-compartment models but in this case the results are far more impressive since an entire spatial pattern of conductance values is produced. The realistic, nonuniform current distributions produced by the model depend on both electrical activity and cell morphology and they develop spontaneously, guided by local intracellular calcium concentrations.

The stability and activity-dependent conductance features found in the single-compartment models were also found in the multi-compartment models, again with the added feature of complex and interesting spatial structure (Siegel, Marder and Abbott, 1994). Different spatial patterns of stimulation produce different conductance distributions. The intrinsic plasticity produced by the activity-dependent distribution of conductances tends to balance the synaptic contribution coming from different dendritic branches. If little synaptic input comes to a particular dendritic branch it may develop enough inward conducances to support action potentials. Activity-dependent regulation can also act as a gain control mechanism to compensate for the effects of long-term potentiation or depression of synapses. This has an important balancing effect on the destabilizing impact of Hebbian synaptic modification, keeping the activity of the neuron in the middle of its range of firing frequencies despite synaptic potentiation. Acting together, intrinsic and synaptic modification produce a system that is highly plastic and yet stable.

4. Experiments

The results of our modeling studies suggest that activity/calcium regulation of maximal conductances has interesting effects on the behavior of model neurons. However, these phenomena only have biological significance if similar activity-dependent modifications of intrinsic properties occur in real neurons. In the modeling studies, our basic thesis was that neurons regulate their conductances not to hold them at fixed values, but rather to maintain a constant average level or pattern of activity. Neurons in the stomatogastric ganglion (STG) of the spiny lobster, *Panulirus interruptus*, have ideal properties for testing this idea in biological rather than model neurons.

The STG generates two rhythmic patterns of activity that drive the teeth and foregut (Harris-Warrick et al., 1992). We will be discussing primarily pyloric neurons of the STG which produce a rhythm with a frequency of around 1 Hz. The rhythmic activity of one pyloric neuron is shown in the left panel of figure 6. This rhythmicity relies on both synaptic connections between STG neurons and on modulatory inputs to the STG from outside the ganglion (Harris-Warrick et al., 1992). Most synapses between pyloric neurons are inhibitory and the neurons fire rebound bursts of action potentials when they are released from inhibition. A crucial feature of these STG neurons for testing our basic thesis is that they do not exhibit rhythmic activity when they are pharmacologically isolated from their synaptic and modulatory inputs. Instead, when pharmacologically isolated they are either silent or they spontaneously fire tonic action potentials, as seen in the right panel of figure 6. Silent isolated neurons will fire action potentials tonically when depolarized by current injection but do not produce rhythmic bursting.

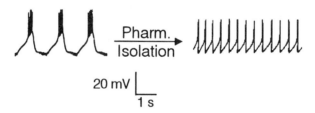

Figure 6: Properties of STG neurons in the ganglion. When connected to their normal synaptic and modulatory inputs in the ganglion these neurons fire in periodic bursts. When pharmacologically isolated from these inputs they either fire tonically or are silent but fire tonically upon depolarization. (Adapted from Turrigiano, Abbott and Marder, 1994.)

The absence of rhythmic bursting in isolated STG neurons indicates that they do not possess the balance of intrinsic conductances needed to generate bursts by themselves. Nevertheless, their normal pattern of activity is to fire in bursts due to synaptic inputs. This leads to a question central to our basic idea: what happens if we isolate STG neurons from their synaptic inputs for a prolonged period of time? The conventional neuronal modeling view would be that the cells should maintain their conductances at constant levels and thus that their properties should not change. If instead the neuron is able to modify its conductances and if it does so in an attempt to maintain a constant level of activity, we should see dramatic changes in the intrinsic properties of chronically isolated STG neurons. Since their normal pattern of activity is bursting, chronically isolated neurons may adjust and modify their conductances in an attempt to restore bursting activity.

To test these ideas we removed STG neurons from the ganglion and studied them individually in primary cell culture (Turrigiano, Abbott and Marder, 1994) using methods discussed by Turrigiano and Marder (1993). The entire neuron cannot be removed from the ganglion during this procedure, only the soma and a short piece of primary neurite are transferred to cell culture. However, over the following few days neurons regrow fairly extensive processes in culture. The issue relevant to this discussion is whether they subsequently retain the same intrinsic properties in culture as they had in the ganglion or whether these change. Furthermore, if intrinsic properties change do they do so in a way consistent with our modeling studies? Specifically, does bursting activity tend to be enhanced through modification of maximal conductances and, if so, does this process rely on intracellular calcium as a feedback element?

5. Experimental Results

After one day in culture, most STG neurons are fairly passive, exhibiting at most weak, damped action potentials upon depolarization. The somata of STG neurons express predominantly outward currents so this initial lack of activity is not surprising. After 2 days in culture, most STG neurons are silent at rest but are able to fire action potentials tonically when they are depolarized or released from hyperpolarization (figure 7, day 2). These properties were similar to those seen in STG neurons pharmacologically isolated in the ganglion (right panel of figure 6). Thus, at this point the neurons appear to have restored the balance of conductances that they had while in the ganglion. However, after 3 or 4 days in culture the majority of STG neurons fire in bursts when depolarized and produce a burst-like slow wave depolarization when they are released from hyperpolarization (figure 7, day 3). Thus, chronically isolated STG neurons do not maintain the intrinsic properties that they had in the ganglion. Instead they modify the balance of their conductances and become capable of generating periodic bursts, at least when depolarized.

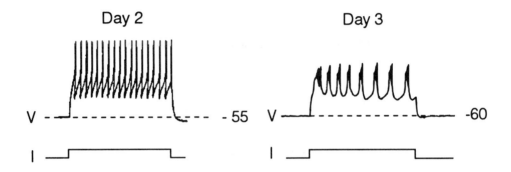

Figure 7: Properties of STG neurons in primary cell culture. Intracellular recordings from STG neurons after 2 and 3 days in culture are shown along with a trace indicating the current injected into them. Typically day 2 neurons fire tonically while day 3 neurons produce burst-like slow-wave oscillations. (Adapted from Turrigiano, Abbott and Marder, 1994.)

The transition from tonic firing to bursting seen in cultured STG neurons is caused by conductance changes similar to those we see in the model neurons. The maximal conductances of inward currents increase during this time period, while outward current maximal conductances decrease (Turrigiano, LeMasson and Marder, 1994). The decrease in outward conductances shows that the neurons are not simply adding active membrane that expresses inward currents while they are growing but are actually regulating their conductances in a more selective manner.

If STG neurons in culture modify their conductances to increase bursting activity, we should be able to affect these modifications by stimulating the neurons. While in the ganglion, STG neurons receive periodic (approximately 0.3-1 Hz for pyloric neurons) inhibition and they fire in bursts when released from this inhibition. This is why they are able to fire rhythmically even though their intrinsic properties do not allow them to generate bursts independently. Can we restore the cultured STG neurons to their original non-bursting state by simulating the periodic input they receive in the ganglion? To answer this question we supplied periodic pulses of hyperpolarizing current through a microelectrode to the cultured STG neurons that

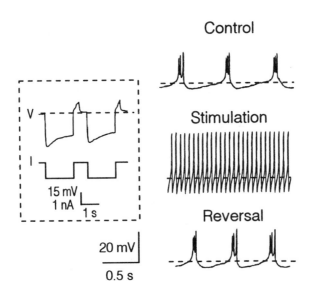

Figure 8: Response of STG neurons to depolarizing current injection before and after 1 hour of rhythmic stimulation. Control: prior to stimulation the neurons exhibited bursting behavior. Stimulation: after 1 hour of hyperpolarizing current pulses the activity changed to tonic firing. Reversal: 1 hour after cessation of current pulses bursting resumed. The insert shows the hyperpolarization and subsequent rebound in response to the injected current pulses. (Adapted from Turrigiano, Abbott and Marder, 1994.)

exhibited intrinsic bursting as in figure 7 on day 3 (figure 8, Control). This simulates the periodic inhibition they receive in the ganglion. The hyperpolarizing pulses caused these neurons to fire bursts on the rebound much as they do in the ganglion (insert of figure 8). After one hour of this stimulation, the response to depolarization changed from bursting to tonic firing as seen in figure 8 (Stimulation). This effect reversed after about one hour without any hyperpolarizing pulses (figure 8, Reversal). Rhythmic drive therefore eliminated the ability of the cultured neuron to burst and restored it to a state similar to what is seen in the ganglion.

Does calcium play a role in the activity-dependent conductance changes seen in the cultured neurons? Several pieces of evidence suggest that it does. We repeated the experiments shown in figure 8 in which period current pulses were delivered to the neurons to reduce or eliminate their bursting properties. In these experiments, after each hyperpolarizing pulse the neurons show a slow-wave depolarization seen in the insert of figure 8 that is blocked by reducing extracellular calcium or by blocking calcium currents. If the same experiment is done on neurons that do not exhibit this slow-wave depolarization or if the rebound depolarization is blocked during the experiment, no activity-dependent changes are observed. This suggests that calcium entry following hyperpolarization plays an essential role in the conductance modification process. Finally, we repeated the type of experiment shown in figure 8 in the presence of bapta, a calcium chelator that buffers the level of intracellular calcium. The presence of bapta completely eliminated the activity-dependent changes in intrinsic properties, again suggesting that a change in the concentration of intracellular calcium is essential. Although calcium plays a crucial role, it is unlikely to be the only relevant factor affecting the activity-dependent changes seen in biological neurons.

6. Discussion

Conductance-based models can simulate the behavior of neurons quite realistically over time scales ranging from milliseconds to seconds. However, over longer time periods from hours to days additional processes involving the synthesis, transport and modulation of ion channels become relevant. These can produce activity-dependent shifts in the intrinsic electrical properties of neurons that, along with synaptic plasticity, are important for network development, stability, adaptation and learning. We have made a start at modeling these slower processes and have found that a number of interesting properties arise:

1. Activity/calcium-regulated model neurons can self-assemble the conductances needed to achieve a desired target electrical activity pattern.

2. When extracellular conditions change, model neurons adjust their maximal conductances to find a new balance of currents that restores the original pattern of activity.

3. The calcium-dependent feedback loop in the model causes the intrinsic properties of model neurons to shift in response to stimulation and to the presence of other neurons in a network.

4. Coupled neurons can differentiate spontaneously so that model neurons described by the same underlying equations can develop different sets of conductances and play different roles in the functioning of a network.

5. A non-uniform distribution of membrane currents can arise in a spatially extended model neuron in response to spatial variations of the intracellular calcium concentration related both to the morphology of the cell and to the pattern of synaptic input it receives.

6. Synaptically driven shifts in the distribution of membrane currents tend to equalize synaptic inputs that are non-uniform over the dendritic tree.

7. Activity-dependent conductances can control the level of excitability of a neuron to compensate for changes in the strengths of its synaptic inputs.

One of the most significant messages provided by models of conductance regulation is that the same mechanisms that develop and maintain membrane conductances are likely to modify these conductances in response to long-lasting changes in the activity of the neuron. Most of the work done on activity-dependent plasticity in networks has focused on synaptic modification. As more is learned about the processes that control channel conductances, activity-dependent plasticity of intrinsic neuronal properties is likely to play an increasing role in understanding network function.

Our modeling studies suggest that neurons do not maintain fixed conductances but rather adjust their conductances in an attempt to maintain a fixed level or pattern of activity and our experimental results support this viewpoint. The data show that patterned input can profoundly alter the intrinsic properties of STG neurons. When these neurons are isolated from rhythmic drive, their ability to burst is enhanced and when rhythmic drive is restored, this ability is reduced or eliminated. This suggests that STG neurons adjust their conductances in an attempt to retain the capacity to fire in bursts despite changes in external inputs and that, in their natural setting within the ganglion, synaptic inputs play a key role in maintaining intrinsic neuronal characteristics.

The activity-dependent process we have discussed require an intracellular feedback element that is well-correlated with electrical activity. We have proposed that intracellular calcium plays this role and our experiments support this idea. Calcium is known to mediate many activity-dependent processes, including changes in synaptic efficacy (Lynch et al., 1983; Madison, Malenka and Nicoll, 1991; Hong and Lnenicka, 1993) and neurite outgrowth (Kater and Mills, 1991; Fields, Neale and Nelson, 1990; Ooyen and van Pelt, 1994) in addition to the magnitude of ionic currents (Alkon, 1984; Franklin, Fickbohm and Willard, 1992; Turrigiano, Abbott and Marder, 1994). This raises the exciting possibility of modeling the development and maintenance of intrinsic neuronal properties, the growth of neuronal circuits and the adjustment of synaptic strengths all through the effects of intracellular calcium.

References

Abbott, L.F. 1994 Single neuron dynamics: An introduction. In Ventriglia, F., ed. Neural Modelling and Neural Networks. Pergamon Press, London. pp. 57-78.

Abbott, L.F. and LeMasson, G. 1993 Analysis of neuron models with dynamically regulated conductances. Neural Comp. Neural Comp. 5:823-842.

Abbott, L.F. and Blum, K.I. 1994 Functional significance of long-term potentiation between hippocampal place cells. (submitted).

Alkon, D.L. 1984 Calcium-mediated reduction of ionic currents: A biophysical memory trace. Science 226:1037-1045.

Armstrong, R.C. and Montminy, M.R. 1993 Transynaptic control of gene expression. Annu. Rev. Neurosci. 16:17-30.

Artola, A. and Singer, W. 1993 Long-term depression of excitatory synaptic transmission and its relationship to long-term potentiation. Trends Neurosci. 16:480-487.

Bell, A. 1992 Self-Organization in real neurons: anti-Hebb in 'channel space'? In Moody, J.E. and Hanson, S.J., eds. Neural Information Processing Systems 4 . Morgan Kaufman, San Mateo CA. pp. 59-66.

Baudry, M. & Davis, J.L., eds. 1991 Long-Term Potentiation. MIT Press, Cambridge MA.

Buchholtz, F., Golowasch, J., Epstein, I. and Marder, E. 1992 Mathematical model of an identified stomatogastric neuron. J. Neurophysiol. 67:332-340.

Byrne, J.H. and Berry W.O. 1989 Neural Models of Plasticity. Academic Press, San Diego.

Chad, J.E. and Eckert, R., 1986, An enzymatic mechanism for calcium current inactivation in dialysed helix neurones, J. Physiol. (London), 378:31-51.

Churchland, P.S. and Sejnowski, T.J. 1992 The Computational Brain. MIT Press, Cambridge, MA.

Fields, R.D., Neale, E.A. and Nelson, P.G. 1990 Effects of patterned electrical activity on neurite outgrowth from mouse neurons. J. Neurosci. 10:2950-2964.

Franklin, J.L., Fickbohm, D.J. and Willard, A.L. 1992 Long-term regulation of neuronal calcium currents by prolonged changes of membrane potential. J. Neurosci. 12:1726-1735.

Gluck, M.A. and Rumelhart, D.E. 1990 Neuroscience and Connectionist Theory. Lawrence Erlbaum, Hillsdale NJ.

Gruol, D.L., Deal, C.R., Yool, A.J. 1992 Developmental changes in calcium conductances contribute to the physiological maturation of cerebellar purkinje neurons in culture. J. Neurosci. 12:2838-2848.

Harris-Warrick R.M. and Marder E. 1991 Modulation of neural networks for behavior. Annu. Rev. Neurosci. 14:39-57.

Harris-Warrick R.M., Marder E., Selverston A.I., Moulins M., Eds. 1992 Dynamic Biological Networks. MIT Press, Cambridge, MA.

Hawkins, R.D., Kandel, E.R. and Siegelbaum, S.A. 1993 Learning to modulate transmitter release: Themes and variations in synaptic plasticity. Annu. Rev. Neurosci. 16:625-665 .

Hemmick, L.M., Perney, T.M., Flamm, R.E., Kaczmarek, L.K. and Birnberg, N.C., 1992, Expression of the h-ras oncogene induces potassium conductance and neuron-specific potassium channel mRNAs in the AtT20 cell line, J. Neurosci., 12:2007-2014.

Hille B. 1992 Ionic Channels of Excitable Membranes. Sinauer Assoc., Sunderland, MA.

Hodgkin A.L., Huxley A.F. 1952 A quantitative description of membrane current and its application to conduction and excitation in nerve. J. Physiol. 117:500-544.

Hong, S.J. and Lnenicka, G.A. 1993 Long-term changes in the neuromuscular synapses of a crayfish motoneuron produced by calcium influx. Brain Res. 605:121-127.

Kaczmarek, L.K. and Levitan, I.B., eds. 1987 Neuromodulation. The Biochemical Control of Neuronal Excitability. Oxford Univ. Press, NY.

Kater, S.B. and Mills, L.R. 1991 Regulation of growth cone behavior by calcium. J. Neurosci. 11:891-899.

Koch, C. and Segev, I., eds. 1989 Methods in Neuronal Modeling. MIT Press, Cambridge MA.

LeMasson, G., Marder, E. and Abbott, L.F. 1993 Activity-dependent regulation of conductances in model neurons. Science 259:1915-1917.

Levy, W.B., Colbert, C.M. and Desmond, N.L. 1990 Elemental adaptive processes of neurons and synapses: a statistical/computational perspective. In Gluck, M.A. and Rumelhart, D.E. eds., Neuroscience and Connectionist Theory. Lawrence Erlbaum, Hillsboro, N.Y. pp. 187-236.

Llinás, R.R. 1988 Intrinsic electrophysiological properties of mammalian neurons: insights into central nervous system function. Science 242:654 -1664.

Lynch, G., Larson, J., Kelso, S., Barrionuevo, G. and Schottler, F. 1983 Intracellular injections of EGTA block induction of hippocampal long-term potentiation. Nature 305:719-721.

Madison, D.V., Malenka, R.C. and Nicoll, R.A. 1991 Mechanisms underlying lont-term potentiation of synaptic transmission. Annu. Rev. Neurosci. 124:379-397.

Malenka, R.C. and Nicoll, R.A. 1993 MBDA-receptor-dependent synaptic plasticity: Multiple forms and mechanisms. Trends Neurosci. 16:521-527.

McCormick, D. A. 1990 Membrane properties and neurotransmitter actions. In Shepherd, G.M., ed. The Synaptic Organization of the Brain. Oxford Univ. Press, New York.

Miller, K.D. 1990 Correlation-based models of neural development. In Gluck, M.A. and Rumelhart, D.E., eds. Neuroscience and Connectionist Theory. Lawrence Erlbaum, Hillsdale NJ. pp. 267-354.

Morgan, J.I., Curran T. 1991 Stimulus-transcription coupling in the nervous system: involvement of the inducible proto-oncogenes fos and jun. Annu. Rev. Neurosci. 14: 421-451.

Morris, C. and Lecar, H. 1981 Voltage oscillations in the barnacle giant muscle fiber. Biophys. J. 35:193-213.

Morris, R.G.M., Anderson, E., Lynch, G.S. and Baudry, M. 1986 Selective impairment of learning and blockade of long-term potentiation by an N-methyl-D-aspartate receptor antagonist, AP5. Nature 319: 774-776.

Murphy, T.H., Worley, P.F., Baraban, J.M. 1991 L-type voltage-sensitive calcium channels mediate synaptic activation of immediate early genes. Neuron 7: 625-635.

Rinzel, J. and Ermentrout, G.B., 1989, Analysis of neural excitability and oscillations In Koch, C. and Segev, I., eds. Methods in Neuronal Modeling. MIT Press, Cambridge MA.

Ross, W.M. 1989 Changes in intracellular calcium during neuron activity. Annu. Rev. Physiol. 51:491-506.

Shatz, J.C.1990 Impulse activity and the patterning of connections during CNS development. Neuron 5:745-756.

Sheng M., Greenberg, M.E. 1990 The regulation and function of c-fos and other immediate early genes in the nervous system. Neuron 4:477-485.

Siegel, M., Marder, E., Abbott, L.F. 1994 Activity-dependent current distributions in model neurons. Proc. Natl. Acad. Sci USA (in press).

Turrigiano, G., Abbott, L.F., Marder, E. 1994 Activity-dependent changes in the intrinsic electrical properties of cultured neurons. Science 264:974-977.

Turrigiano, G. LeMasson, G. and Marder, E. 1994 Selective regulation of current densities underlies spontaneous changes in the activity of cultured neurons. (submitted).

Turrigiano, G. and Marder, E. 1993 Modulation of identified stomatogastric ganglion neurons in primary cell culture. J. Neurophysiol. 69:1993-2001.

van Ooyen, A. and van Pelt, J. 1994 Activity-dependent outgrowth of neurons and overshoot phenomenoa in developing neural networks. J. Theor. Biol. 167:27-44.

Research supported by National Institutes of Health grants MH46742 and NS17813 and National Science Foundation grant DMS-9208206. G. LeMasson is currently at Laboratoire de Neurobiologie et Physiologie Comparées, Place du Dr. Peyneau, 33120 Arcachon, France.

Chapter 4
Evolution of Parallel Processes
in Organic and Digital Media*

Thomas S. Ray†

Abstract

Life can be thought of as an information process, in which the programs being run are the genomes of living organisms. The individual cells can be thought of as the processors. There are many cell types in large organisms, and different cell types express different genes (execute different code), while cells of the same type express the same genes. Thus multi-cellular organisms exhibit parallelism on an astronomical scale, as there are trillions of cells in large organisms. These organisms are parallel processes exhibiting both SIMD and MIMD parallelism, integrated into beautifully coordinated systems. Evolution is the process that created this genetic software embedded in wetware, and initial experiments demonstrate that evolution can operate effectively with machine code software embedded in hardware. This paper describes an approach for using the evolutionary process to generate complex parallel processes embedded in massively parallel or distributed computational systems.

1 Introduction

The process of evolution by natural selection is able to create complex and beautiful information processing systems (such as· primate nervous systems) without the guidance of an intelligent supervisor. Yet intelligent programmers have not been able to produce software systems that match even the capabilities of primitive organisms such as insects. Recent experiments demonstrate that evolution by natural selection is able to

*This work was supported by grants CCR-9204339 and BIR-9300800 from the United States National Science Foundation, a grant from the Digital Equipment Corporation, and by the Santa Fe Institute, Thinking Machines Corp., IBM, and Hughes Aircraft. This work was conducted while at: ATR, Japan; Biology Department, University of Delaware, Newark, Delaware, 19716, USA; and Santa Fe Institute, 1660 Old Pecos Trail, Suite A, Santa Fe, New Mexico, 87501, USA.

†ATR Human Information Processing Research Laboratories, 2-2 Hikaridai, Seika-cho, Soraku-gun, Kyoto, 619-02, Japan, ray@hip.atr.co.jp, ray@santafe.edu, ray@udel.edu

operate effectively in genetic languages based on the machine codes of digital computers [12, 15, 20]. This opens up the possibility of using evolution to generate complex software.

Through iterated replication-with-selection of large populations through many generations, evolution by natural selection searches out the possibilities inherent in the "physics and chemistry" of the medium in which it is embedded. It exploits any inherent self-organizing properties of the medium, and flows into natural attractors realizing and fleshing out their structure.

Evolution never escapes from its ultimate imperative: self-replication. However, the mechanisms that evolution discovers for achieving this ultimate goal gradually become so convoluted and complex that the underlying drive can seem to become superfluous. Evolution is both a defining characteristic and the creative process of life itself. The living condition is a state that complex physical systems naturally flow into under certain conditions. It is a self-organizing, self-perpetuating state of auto-catalytically increasing complexity. The living component of the physical system quickly becomes the most complex part of the system, such that it re-shapes the medium, in its own image as it were. Life then evolves adaptations predominantly in relation to the living components of the system, rather than the non-living components. Life evolves adaptations to itself.

Until recently, life has been known as a state of matter, particularly combinations of the elements carbon, hydrogen, oxygen, nitrogen and smaller quantities of many others. However, recent work in the field of Artificial Life has shown that the natural evolutionary process can proceed with great efficacy in other media, such as the informational medium of the digital computer [6, 12, 13, 14, 15, 16, 17, 19, 20]

These new natural evolutions, in artificial media, are beginning to explore the possibilities inherent in the "physics and chemistry" of those media. They are organizing themselves and constructing self-generating complex systems. While these new living systems are still so young that they remain in their primordial state, it appears that they have embarked on the same kind of journey taken by life on earth, and presumably have the potential to evolve levels of complexity that could lead to sentient and eventually intelligent beings.

Here I am discussing the possibility that evolution in the digital medium could produce information processes of vastly greater complexity than any digital processes in existance today. Possibly, digital evolution could produce processes approaching or rivaling the functionality of the human brain. While such a suggestion seems fantastic, it is based on a metaphor between evolution in the digital and in the organic media. In the medium of carbon chemistry, evolution apparently began with simple self-replicating molecules, and caused the complexity of the replicating structures to increase by many orders of magnitude.

Initial experiments described below, indicate that evolution by natural selection also works effectively in the digital medium. This raises the question of how far digital evolution can go in increasing the complexity of its replicators? We don't know the answer to this question, and can only find out through experimentation. The main objective of this paper is to suggest an approach for guiding experimentation aimed at provoking digital evolution to generate large increases in the complexity of its replicators.

The bulk of this manuscript consists of suggesting directions, methodologies and a philosophy for research on the potential of evolution in generating complexity in the digital medium. As such, it discusses mostly ideas, not results. These ideas are discussed in an air of optimistic and unhibited consideration of the possibilities for digital evolution. However, let it be said that I am a pragmatist and consider results to be the bottom line. I am charting a research direction that I consider to be worth exploring. In fact the potential rewards are so great that I consider it imperative to make the attempt. However, I am not prepared to speculate on the probability of success. Let us make the experiments, and the results will speak for themselves.

2   The Approach

The objective of the approach discussed here, is to create an instantiation of evolution by natural selection in the computational medium. This creates a conceptual problem that requires considerable art to solve: ideas and techniques must be learned by studying organic evolution, and then applied to the generation of evolution in a digital medium, without forcing the digital medium into an "un-natural" simulation of the organic world.

We must derive inspiration from observations of organic life, but we must never lose sight of the fact that the new instantiation is not organic, and may differ in many fundamental ways. For example, organic life inhabits a Euclidean space, however computer memory is not a Euclidean space. Inter-cellular communication in the organic world is chemical in nature, and therefore a single message generally can pass no more information than on or off. By contrast, communication in digital computers generally involves the passing of bit patterns, which can carry much more information.

The fundamental principal of the approach being advocated here is *to understand and respect the natural form of the digital computer, to facilitate the process of evolution in generating forms that are adapted to the computational medium, and to let evolution find forms and processes that naturally exploit the possibilities inherent in the medium.*

Situations arise where it is necessary to make significant changes from the standard computer architecture. But such changes should be made with caution, and only when there is some feature of standard computer architectures which clearly inhibits the desired processes.

3   Experimental Methods

The methodology has been described in detail [6, 12, 13, 14, 15, 17], so it will be described only briefly here. The software used in this study is available over the net or on disk (contact the author). A new set of computer architectures has been designed which have the feature that their machine code is robust to the genetic operations of mutation and recombination. This means that computer programs written in the machine code of these architectures remain viable some of the time after being randomly altered by bit-flips which cause the swapping of individual instructions with others from within the instruction set, or by swapping segments of code between programs (through a spontaneous sexual process). These new computers have not been built in silicon, but exist only as software prototypes known as "virtual computers". These virtual computers have been called "Tierra", Spanish for Earth.

A self-replicating program was written, initially in Intel machine language. This program was then implemented in the first of the Tierran languages in the fall of 1989. The program functions by examining itself to determine where it begins and ends, then calculating its size (80 bytes), and then copying itself one byte at a time to another location in memory. After that, both programs replicate, and the number of programs "living" in memory doubles in each generation.

These programs are referred to as "creatures" or "organisms". The creatures occupy a finite amount of memory called the "soup". The operating system of the virtual computer, Tierra, provides services to allocate CPU time to the growing population of self-replicating creatures. When the creatures fill the soup, the operating system invokes a "reaper" facility which kills creatures to insure that memory will remain free for occupation by newborn creatures. Thus a turnover of generations of individuals begins when the memory is full.

The operating system also generates a variety of errors which play the role of mutations. One kind of error is a bit-flip, in which a zero is converted to a one, or a one is converted to a zero. This occurs in the soup, which is where the "genetic" information that constitutes the programs of the creatures resides. The bit-flips are the analogs of mutations, and cause swapping among the thirty-two instructions of the machine code. Another kind of error imposed by the operating system is called a "flaw", in which calculations taking place within the CPU of the virtual machine may be inaccurate, or in which any transfer of information may move information to or from the wrong place, or may slightly alter information in transit.

The machine code that makes up the program of a creature is the analog of the genome, the DNA, of organic creatures. Mutations cause genetic change and are therefore heritable. Flaws do not directly cause genetic change, and so are not heritable. However, flaws may cause errors in the *process* of self-replication, resulting in offspring which are genetically different from their parents, and those differences are then heritable.

The running of the self-replicating program (creature) on the virtual computer (Tierra), with the errors imposed by the operating system (mutations) results in precisely the conditions described by Darwin as causing evolution by natural selection. While this is actually an instantiation of Darwinian evolution in a digital medium, it can also be viewed as a metaphor: The sequence of machine instructions that constitute the program of a creature is analogous to the sequence of nucleotides that constitute the genome, the DNA, of organic organisms. The soup, a block of RAM memory of the computer, is thought of as the spatial resource. The CPU time provided by the virtual computer is thought of as the energy resource. The sequences of machine instructions that make up the genomes of the creatures constitute an informational resource which plays an important role in evolution.

4 Experimental Results

Diverse ecological communities have emerged. These digital communities have been used to experimentally examine ecological and evolutionary processes: e.g., competitive exclusion and coexistence, host/parasite density dependent population regulation, the effect of parasites in enhancing community diversity, evolutionary races, punctuated equilibrium, and the role of chance and historical factors in evolution.

From a single rudimentary ancestral "creature" there have evolved tens of thousands of self-replicating genotypes of many hundreds of genome size classes. Bit flipping mutations cause changes in the sequence of instructions in the genome, but they do not cause changes in the size of the genome. However, mutant genotypes make errors in their self-examination and replication, resulting in different sized genomes. As genetic change generates new genotypes, variants appear which are able to replicate more rapidly than their ancestors, and those variants increase in frequency in the soup.

Very quickly there evolve parasites, which are not able to replicate in isolation because they lack a large portion of the genome. However, these parasites search for the missing information, and if they locate it in a nearby creature, they parasitize the information from the neighboring genome, thereby effecting their own replication. This informational parasitism is a commensal relationship, as it is not directly detrimental to the host. However, the parasites do compete with the hosts for space, and may be superior competitors because they can more rapidly replicate their smaller genome. However, their advantage is frequency dependent. As the parasites increase in frequency, the hosts decline, and many parasites fail to locate hosts. In ecological runs, without genetic change, hosts and parasites demonstrate Lotka-Volterra cycles.

In some runs, hosts evolve immunity to attack by parasites. One immune mechanism that has been worked out is based on the fact that the creatures only examine themselves once, and rely on retaining the information on their size and location for all subsequent replications. Immune hosts cause their parasites to loose their sense of self by failing to retain the information on size and location. Immune hosts function with this forgetful code by re-examining themselves before each replication, thus there is a metabolic cost to the immunity.

When immune hosts appear, they often increase in frequency, devastating the parasite populations. In some runs where the community comes to be dominated by immune hosts, parasites evolve that are resistant to immunity. The above mentioned immune mechanism can by circumvented by parasites which also re-examine themselves before each replication.

Hosts sometimes evolve a response to parasites that goes beyond immunity to actual hyper-parasitism. Hyper-parasites allow themselves to be parasitized, letting the parasite use their code for a single replication. After the first replication, the hyper-parasite deceives the parasite by replacing the parasite's record of its size and location with the size and location of the hyper-parasite genome. Thereafter, the parasite will devote its energetic resources to replication of the hyper-parasite genome. This is a highly deleterious interaction, which drives the parasites to extinction. The hyper-parasites are facultative, getting an energy boost when the parasites are present, but not requiring them for replication.

Evolving in the absence of parasites, hyper-parasites completely dominate the community, resulting in a relatively uniform community characterize by a high degree of relationship between individuals. Under these circumstances, sociality evolves, in the sense that the creatures evolve into forms which can not replicate in isolation, but which can only replicate in aggregations. These colonial creatures cooperate in the control of the flow of execution of their algorithms.

The cooperative behavior of the social hyper-parasites makes them vulnerable to a new class of parasites. These cheaters, hyper-hyper-parasites, insert themselves between cooperating social individuals, and momentarily seize control of execution of the algorithm, just long enough to deceive the social creatures about their size and location, causing the social creatures to replicate the genomes of the cheaters.

In a separate experiment, two versions of the ancestral creature were made, each with a different portion of the genome deleted. Neither of these genomes were able to replicate in isolation. However, when cultured together, they each parasitize the missing code from the other, forming an ecologically stable obligate symbiotic relationship. When genetic change is allowed in the symbiotic system, a very complex series of changes follows, ultimately resulting in the merging of the two genomes into a single self-replicating genome.

One of the most interesting aspects of digital life is that the bulk of the evolution is based on adaptation to the living environment rather than the physical environment. It is co-evolution that drives the system.

The only kind of genetic change that the simulator imposes on the system is random bit flips in the machine code of the creatures. However, it turns out that parasites are very sloppy replicators. They cause significant recombination and rearrangement of the genomes. This spontaneous sexuality is a powerful force for evolutionary change in the system.

A series of experiments were conducted on the effects of mutation rates on the rates of evolution [15]. The parameter used to compare rates of evolution was the rate at which self-replicating genomes decreased in size, indicating an optimization, in an environment favoring smaller sizes. The optimal mutation rate was found to be a mutation affecting one in four individuals per generation. At higher rates the community sometimes died out, as genomes melted under the mutational heat. At lower rates, optimization was slower. Fully self-replicating (non-parasitic) genomes reduced from 80 instructions to as few as 22 instructions overnight (more than 1500 generations, of populations ranging from 300 to 1000) individuals. The ancestor of size 80 requires 839 CPU cycles to replicate. The creature of size 22 requires 146 CPU cycles to replicate, a 5.75-fold difference in efficiency.

However, not all evolutionary optimizations were achieved through production of the most compact algorithm. Some solutions involved the evolution of more complex algorithms that achieved optimization through efficiency rather than size [20]. These algorithms utilized the technique of "unrolling the loop", which requires more code. Some of these repeated the work two times, and others three times, within the loop. These solutions require more intricate algorithms than the one found in the ancestral algorithm, and illustrate the capacity of evolution to generate increasingly complex structures.

A comparison was made of the patterns of evolution in four different machine instruction sets [20]. These instruction sets vary in the way that information is moved among the registers of the CPU, and the way that the registers are addressed. There were striking differences in the mode and degree of evolution in the four sets. Two sets show gradualism, one punctuated equilibrium, and one punctuated gradualism. Those exhibiting punctuations achieve greater degrees of evolution.

The relationship between evolution and entropy has been studied by measuring entropy as genetic diversity in the soup ($-\sum p \log p$, where p is the proportion of the soup occupied by a genotype class) [20]. This measure of entropy rises rapidly to an equilibrium value, where it remains thereafter, drifting slowly upwards (probably due to an increase in the population due to the decreasing size of individuals). However, there are occasional sharp drops in entropy, corresponding to episodes of extinction. These extinction episodes are not provoked by external perturbations, but are internally generated.

The extinction episodes generally correspond the the origin of some new and very successful mode of existence, which causes the originating genotype to increase rapidly in population, driving other genotypes to extinction. This often occurs when parasites evolve a means of circumventing the immune mechanisms of the hosts. However, the descendents of the new successful genotype rapidly diversify restoring the community to the equilibrium entropy.

Some initial experiments with the evolution of parallel processes have recently been conducted [21]. In these experiments, the standard Tierran self-replicating ancestor was parallelized. The instruction set was enhanced by the inclusion of **split** and **join** instructions, so that new processes could be spawned and terminated by individual organisms. The soup was then seeded with an ancestor which spawned a second process, and divided the work of copying the genome between these two processors, such that one processor copied the first half of the genome while the second processor copied the second half of the genome.

When this organism was allowed to evolve, its descendants learned to spawn two additional processes, and divide the work of copying the genome evenly between the four processors. This higher level of parallelism required some additional computation in preparation for the parallel phase of the algorithm, to coordinate the activity of the additional processors. Therefore the more parallel algorithm was also a more complex algorithm, but one which gained in efficiency through additional parallelism. Organisms have evolved to use up to sixteen processors (the allowed limit), and have distributed the work perfectly among the processors, even when the work does not divide evenly by the number of processors.

These experiments have demonstrated that evolution can work effectively with the mechanisms of parallel computation, yet they are only a first step along a long road. The parallelism evolved in this experiment is still essentially of the SIMD kind, in that each processor is executing the same code, but operating on different data. The next step is to evolve MIMD style programming.

5   The Computational Medium

The computational medium of the digital computer is an informational universe of boolean logic, not a material one. Digital organisms live in the memory of the computer, and are powered by the activity of the central processing unit (CPU). Whether the hardware of the CPU and memory is built of silicon chips, vacuum tubes, magnetic cores, or mechanical switches is irrelevant to the digital organism. Digital organisms should be able to take on the same form in any computational hardware implementing the same logic.

Digital organisms might as well live in a different universe from us, as they are not subject to the same laws of physics and chemistry. They are subject to the "physics and chemistry" of the rules governing the manipulation of bits and bytes within the computer's memory and CPU. They never "see" the actual material from which the computer is constructed, they see only the logic and rules of the CPU and the operating system. These rules are the only "natural laws" that govern their behavior. They are not influenced by the natural laws that govern the material universe (e.g., the laws of thermodynamics).

A typical instantiation of this type involves the introduction of a self-replicating machine language program into the RAM memory of a computer subject to random errors such as bit flips in the memory or occasionally inaccurate calculations [1, 2, 5, 9, 12]. This generates the basic conditions for evolution by natural selection as outlined by Darwin [3]: self-replication in a finite environment with heritable genetic variation.

In this instantiation, the self-replicating machine language program is thought of as the individual "digital organism" or "creature". The RAM memory provides the physical space that the creatures occupy. The CPU provides the source of energy. The memory consists of a large array of bits, generally grouped into eight bit bytes and sixteen or thirty-two bit words. Information is stored in these arrays as voltage patterns which we usually symbolize as patterns of ones and zeros.

The "body" of a digital organism is the information pattern in memory that constitutes its machine language program. This information pattern is data, but when it is passed to the CPU, it is interpreted as a series of executable instructions. These instructions are arranged in such a way that the data of the body will be copied to another location of memory. The informational patterns stored in the memory are altered only through the activity of the CPU. It is for this reason that the CPU is thought of as the analog of the energy source. Without the activity of the CPU, the memory would be static, with no changes in the informational patterns stored there.

The instruction set of the CPU, the memory, and the operating system together define the complete "physics and chemistry" of the universe inhabited by the digital organism. They constitute the physical environment within which digital organisms will evolve. Evolving digital organisms will compete for access to the limited resources of memory space and CPU time, and evolution will generate adaptations for the more agile access to and the more efficient use of these resources.

6   The Living Environment

Some rain forests in the Amazon region occur on white sand soils. In these locations, the physical environment consists of clean white sand, air, falling water, and sunlight. Embedded within this relatively simple physical context we find one of the most complex ecosystems on earth, containing hundreds of thousands of species. These species do not represent hundreds of thousands of adaptations to the physical environment. Most of the adaptations of these species are to the other living organism. The forest creates its own environment.

Life is an auto-catalytic process that builds on itself. Ecological communities are complex webs of species, each living off of others, and being lived off of by others. The system is self-constructing, self-perpetuating, and feeds on itself. Living organisms interface with the non-living physical environment, exchanging materials with it, such as oxygen, carbon-dioxide, nitrogen, and various minerals. However, in the richest ecosystems, the living components of the environment predominate over the physical components.

With living organisms constituting the predominant features of the environment, the evolutionary process is primarily concerned with adaptation to the living environment. Thus ecological interactions are an important driving force for evolution. Species evolve adaptations to exploit other species (to eat them, to parasitize them, to climb on them, to nest on them, to catch a ride on them, etc.) and to defend against such exploitation where it creates a burden.

This situation creates an interesting dynamic. Evolution is predominantly concerned with creating and maintaining adaptations to living organisms which are themselves evolving. This generates evolutionary races among groups of species that interact ecologically. These races can catalyze the evolution of upwardly spiraling complexity as each species evolves to overcome the adaptations of the others. Imagine for example, a predator and prey, each evolving to increase its speed and agility, in capturing prey, or in evading capture. This coupled evolutionary race can lead to increasingly complex nervous systems in the evolving predator and prey species.

What this discussion points to is the importance of embedding evolving synthetic organisms into a context in which they may interact with other evolving organisms. A counter example is the standard implementations of genetic algorithms in which the evolving entities interact only with the fitness function, and never "see" the other entities in the population. Many interesting behavioral, ecological and evolutionary phenomena can only emerge from interactions among the evolving entities.

7 Multi-cellularity

Multi-celled digital organisms are parallel processes. By attempting to synthesize multi-celled digital organisms we can simultaneously explore the biological issues surrounding the evolutionary transition from single-celled to multi-celled life, and the computational issues surrounding the design of complex parallel software.

7.1 Biological Perspective — Cambrian Explosion

Life appeared on earth somewhere between three and four billion years ago. While the origin of life is generally recognized as an event of the first order, there is another event in the history of life that is less well known but of comparable significance. The origin of biological diversity and at the same time of complex macroscopic multi-cellular life, occurred abruptly in the Cambrian explosion 600 million years ago. This event involved a riotous diversification of life forms. Dozens of phyla appeared suddenly, many existing only fleetingly, as diverse and sometimes bizarre ways of life were explored in a relative ecological void [7, 11].

The Cambrian explosion was a time of phenomenal and spontaneous increase in the complexity of living systems. It was the process initiated at this time that led to the evolution of immune systems, nervous systems, physiological systems, developmental systems, complex morphology, and complex ecosystems. To understand the Cambrian explosion is to understand the evolution of complexity. If the history of organic life can be used as a guide, the transition from single celled to multi-celled organisms should be critical in achieving a rich diversity and complexity of synthetic life forms.

7.2 Computational Perspective — Parallel Processes

There already exist a variety of parallel hardware platforms, but our ability to fully utilize the potential of these machines is constrained by our inability to write software of a sufficient complexity. There are two fairly distinctive kinds of parallel architecture in use today: SIMD (single instruction multiple data) and MIMD (multiple instruction multiple data). In the SIMD architecture, the machine may have thousands of processors, but in each CPU cycle, all of the processors must execute the same instruction, although they may operate on different data. It is relatively easy to write software for this kind of machine, since what is essentially a normal sequential program will be broadcast to all the processors.

In the MIMD architecture, there exists the capability for each of the hundreds or thousands of processors to be executing different code, but to have all of that activity coordinated on a common task. However, there does not exist an art for writing this kind of software, at least not on a scale involving more than a few parallel processes. In fact it seems unlikely that human programmers will ever be capable of actually writing software of such complexity.

7.3 Evolution as a Proven Route

It is generally recognized that evolution is the only process with a proven ability to generate intelligence. It is less well recognized that evolution also has a proven ability to generate parallel software of great complexity. In making life a metaphor for computation we will think of the genome, the DNA, as the program, and we will think of each cell in the organism as a processor (CPU). A large multi-celled organism like a human contains trillions of cells/processors.   The genetic program contains billions of nucleotides/instructions.

In a multi-celled organism, cells are differentiated into many cell types such as brain cells, muscle cells, liver cells, kidney cells, etc. The cell types just named are actually general classes of cell types within which there are many sub-types. However, when we specify the ultimate indivisible types, what characterizes a type is the set of genes it expresses. Different cell types express different combinations of genes. In a large organism, there will be a very large number of cells of most types. All cells of the same type express the same genes.

The cells of a single cell type can be thought of as exhibiting parallelism of the SIMD kind, as they are all running the same "program" by expressing the same genes.   Cells of different cell types exhibit MIMD parallelism as they run different code by expressing different genes. Thus large multi-cellular organisms display parallelism on an astronomical scale, combining both SIMD and MIMD parallelism into a beautifully integrated whole. From these considerations it is evident that evolution has a proven ability to generate massively parallel software embedded in wetware. The computational goal of evolving multi-cellular digital organisms is to produce such software embedded in hardware.

7.4 Digital "Neural Networks" — Natural Artificial Intelligence

One of the greatest challenges in the field of computer science is to produce computer systems that are "intelligent" in some way. This might involve for example, the creation of a system for the guidance of a robot which is capable of moving freely in a complex environment, seeking, recognizing and manipulating a variety of objects. It might involve the creation of a system capable of communicating with humans in natural spoken human language, or of translating between human languages. It might be intelligent autonomous agents navigating the internet, seeing out information that we have requested.

It has been observed that natural systems with these capabilities are controlled by nervous systems consisting of large numbers of neurons interconnected by axons and dendrites. Borrowing from nature, a great deal of work has gone into setting up "neural networks" in computers [4, 8]. In these systems, a collection of simulated "neurons" are created, and connected so that they can pass messages. The learning that takes place is accomplished by adjusting the "weights" of the connections.

Organic neurons are essentially analog devices, thus neural networks are implemented on computers as digital emulations of analog devices. There is a certain inefficiency involved in emulating an analog device on a digital computer. For this reason, specialized analog hardware has been developed for the more efficient implementation of artificial neural nets [10].

Neural networks, as implemented in computers, either digital or analog, are intentional mimics of organic nervous systems. They are designed to function like natural neural networks in many details. However, natural neural networks represent the solution found by evolution to the problem of creating an information processing system based on organic chemistry. Evolution works with the physics and chemistry of the medium in which it is embedded.

The solution that evolution found to the problem of communication between organic cells is chemical. Cells communicate by releasing chemicals that bind to and activate receptor molecules on target cells. Working within this medium, evolution created neural nets. Inter-cellular chemical communication in neural nets is "digital" in the sense that chemical messages are either present or not present (on or off). In this sense, a single chemical message carries only a single bit of information. More detailed information can be derived from the temporal pattern of the messages, and also the context of the message. The context can include where on the target cell body the message is applied (which influences its "weight"), and what other messages are arriving at the same time, with which the message in question will be integrated.

It is hoped that evolving multi-cellular digital organisms will become very complex, and will contain some kind of control system that fills the functional role of the nervous system. While it seems likely that the digital nervous system would consist of a network of communicating "cells", it seem unlikely that this would bear much resemblance to conventional neural networks.

Compare the mechanism of inter-cellular communication in organic cells (described above), to the mechanisms of inter-process communication in computers. Processes transmit messages in the form of bit patterns, which may be of any length, and so which may contain any amount of information. Information need not be encoded into the temporal pattern of impulse trains. This and other fundamental differences in communication mechanisms between the digital and the organic media must influence the course that evolution will take as it creates information processing systems in the two media.

It seems highly unlikely that evolution in the digital context would produce information processing systems that would use the same forms and mechanisms as natural neural nets (e.g., weighted connections, integration of incoming messages, threshold triggered all or nothing output, thousands of connections per unit). The organic medium is a physical/chemical medium, whereas the digital medium is a logical/informational medium. That observation alone would suggest that the digital medium is better suited to the construction of information processing systems.

If this is true, then it may be possible to produce digitally based systems that have functionality equivalent to natural neural networks, but which have a much greater simplicity of structure and process. Given evolution's ability to discover the possibilities inherent in a medium, and it's complete lack of preconceptions, it would be very interesting to observe what kind of information processing systems evolution would construct in the digital medium. If evolution is capable of creating network based information processing systems, it may provide us with a new paradigm for digital "connectionism", that would be more natural to the digital medium than simulations of natural neural networks.

8   Making a Digital Cambrian Explosion on the Global Network

Ideally we would like to generate software that utilizes the full capability of our most advanced hardware, particularly massively parallel and networked computational systems. Yet it remains an open question if evolution has the ability to achieve such complexity in the computational medium, and if it does, how that goal can be achieved. Successful efforts at the evolution of machine codes have generally worked with programs of under a hundred bytes. How can we provoke evolution to transform such simple algorithms into software of vast complexity?

Perhaps we can gain some clues to solving this problem by studying the comparable evolutionary transformation in organic life forms: the Cambrian explosion of diversity and complexity. At that point in time, life made an abrupt transformation from simple microscopic single celled forms lacking nervous systems, to large and complex multi-celled forms with nervous systems capable of coordinating sophisticated behavior.

It is heartening to observe that once conditions are right, evolution can achieve extremely rapid increases in complexity and diversity, generating sophisticated information processing systems where previously none existed. However, our problem is to engineer the proper conditions for digital organisms in order to place them on the threshold of a digital version of the Cambrian explosion. Otherwise we might have to wait millions of years to achieve our goal. Ray [17] has reviewed the biological issues surrounding the evolution of diversity and complexity, and they lead to the following conclusions:

Evolution of complexity in the organic world occured in the context of an ecological community of interacting evolving species. Such communities need large complex spaces to exist. A large and complex environment consisting of partially isolated habitats differing and occasionally changing in environmental conditions would be the most conducive to a rapid increase in diversity and complexity.

These are the considerations that lead to the suggestion of the creation of a large and complex ecological reserve for digital organisms. Due to its size, topological complexity, and dynamically changing form and conditions, the global network of computers appears to be an ideal habitat for the evolution of complex digital organisms.

The Tierra system creates a virtual computer (a software emulation of a computer that has not been built in hardware) whose architecture, instruction set, and operating system have been designed to support the evolution of the machine code programs that execute on that virtual machine. A network version of the Tierra system is under development that will allow the passage of messages between Tierra systems installed on different machines connected to the network, via "sockets".

The instruction sets of the Tierran virtual computers will have some new instructions added that allow the digital organisms to communicate between themselves, both within a single installation of Tierra, and over the net between two or more installations. The digital organisms will be able to pass messages consisting of bit strings, and will also be able to send their genomes (their executable code) over the network between installations of Tierra.

The network installation of Tierra will create a virtual sub-network within which digital organisms will be able to move and communicate freely. This network will have a complex topology of interconnections, reflecting the topology of the internet within which it is embedded. In addition, there will be complex patterns of "energy availability" (availability of CPU cycles) due to the Tierra installations being run as low priority background processes and the heterogeneous nature of the real hardware connected to the net. A miniature version of this concept has already been implemented in the form of a CM5 version of Tierra, which will be used to simulate the network version [21].

Consider that each node on the net tends to experience a daily cycle of activity, reflecting the habits of the user who works at that node. The availability of CPU time to the Tierra process will mirror the activity of the user, as Tierra will get only the cycles not required by the user for other processes. Statistically, there will tend to be more "energy" available for the digital organisms at night, when the users are sleeping. However, this will depend a great deal on the habits of the individual users and will vary from day to day.

There will be strong selective pressures for digital organisms to maintain themselves on nodes with a high availability of energy. To a first approximation, this will involve daily migrations around the planet, keeping on the dark side. However, they need to evolve some direct sensory capabilities in order to respond to local deviations from the expected patterns. When rich energy resources are detected on a local sub-net, it may be advantageous to disperse locally within the sub-net, rather than to disperse long distances. Thus there is likely to be selection to control the "directionality" and distances of movement within the net.

All of these conditions should encourage the evolution of "sensory" capabilities to detect energy conditions and spatial structure on the net, and also evolution of the ability to detect temporal patterns in these same features. In addition to the ability to detect these patterns, the digital organisms need the ability to coordinate their actions and movements in response to changing conditions. In short, the digital organisms must be able to intelligently navigate the net in response to the dynamically changing circumstances.

A primary obstacle to the evolution of complexity in the Tierra system has been that in the relatively simple single node installation, a very simple twenty to forty byte algorithm that quickly and efficiently copies itself can not be beat by a much more complex algorithm, which due to its greater size would take much longer to replicate. There is just no need to do anything more complicated than copy yourself quickly. However, the heterogeneous and changing patterns of energy availability and network topology of the network version will reward more complex behavior. It is hoped that this will launch evolution in the direction of more complexity. Once this trajectory has begun, the interactions among the increasingly sophisticated organisms themselves should lead to further complexity increases.

It is imagined that individual digital organisms will be multi-celled, and that the cells that constitute an individual will be dispersed over the net. The remote cells might play a sensory function, relaying information about energy levels around the net back to some "central nervous system" where the incoming sensory information can be processed and decisions made on appropriate actions. If there are some massively parallel machines participating in the virtual net, digital organisms may choose to deploy their central nervous systems on these arrays of tightly coupled processors.

9 "Managing" Evolution

Some questions frequently asked about software evolution are: How can we guide evolution to produce useful application software? How can we validate the code produced by evolution to be sure that it performs the application correctly? These questions reveal a limited view of how software evolution can be used, and what it can be used for. I will articulate a fairly radical view here.

Evolution would not be an appropriate technique for generating accounting software, or any software where precise and accurate computations are required. Evolution would be more appropriate for more fuzzy problems like pattern recognition. For example, if you get a puppy that you want to raise to be a guard dog, you can't verify the neural circuitry or the genetic code, but you can tell if it learns to bark at strangers and is friendly to your family and friends. This is the type of application that evolution can deliver. We don't need to verify the code, but verification of the performance should be straightforward.

Furthermore, attempts to guide early evolution towards a desired application are likely to inhibit its creative potential. Once evolution by natural selection has already produced an incipient application, then guidance through artificial selection (breeding) can enhance the quality of the application. However, we should not attempt to guide evolution to generate the application in the first place. Instead, we should wait to see what evolution offers us. After all, we don't necessarily know what we want.

Computer magazines bemoan the search for the "next killer application", some category of software that everybody will want, but which nobody has thought of yet. The markets for the existing major applications (word processors, spread sheets, data bases, etc.) are already saturated. Growth of the software industry depends on inventing completely new applications. This implies that there are categories of software that everyone will want but which haven't been invented yet. We need not attempt to use evolution to produce superior versions of existing applications. Rather we should allow evolution to find the new applications for us. To see this process more clearly, consider how we manage applications through organic evolution.

Some of the applications provided by organic evolution are: rice, corn, wheat, carrots, beef cattle, dairy cattle, pigs, chickens, dogs, cats, guppies, cotton, mahogany, tobacco, mink, sheep, silk moths, yeast, and penicillin mold. If we had never encountered any one of these organisms, we would never have thought of them either. We have made them into applications because we recognized the potential in some organism that was spontaneously generated within an ecosystem of organisms evolving freely by natural selection.

If the silk moth never existed, but we somehow came up with a complete description of silk, it would be futile to attempt the guide the evolution of any existing creature to produce silk. It is much more productive to survey the bounty of organisms already generated by evolution with an eye to spotting new applications for existing organisms. Some breeding may be necessary to make the application practical. For example, corn, dogs, and cattle are all highly bred organisms, of much greater utility in their present form than that of their wild ancestors.

Imagine for a moment that a team of earth biologists had arrived at a planet at the moment of the initiation of its Cambrian explosion of diversity. Suppose that these biologists came with a list of the application organisms listed above (rice, corn, etc.), and a complete description of each. Could those biologists intervene in the evolutionary process to hasten the production of any of those organisms? Not only is that unlikely, but any attempts to intervene in the process are like to inhibit the diversification itself.

It is preposterous to suppose that humans could guide the evolution of useful complex organisms from their simple single celled ancestors. In fact, we couldn't even imagine what the possibilities are, much less know how to reach those possibilities if we could conceive of them. Fortunately, our intervention is not necessary. Evolution by natural selection will produce a wealth of complex organisms, and we can survey them and bring those with potential uses into breeding and domestication programs.

10   A Better Medium

Natural evolution in the digital medium is a new technology, about which we know very little. The hope is to evolve software with sophisticated functionality far beyond anything that has been designed by humans. But how long might this take? Evolution in the organic medium is known to be a slow process. Certainly there remains the possibility that evolution in the digital medium will be too slow to be a practical tool for software generation, but several observations can be made that provide encouragement.

First, computational processes occur at electronic speeds, and are in fact relatively fast. Second, as was noted above, during the Cambrian explosion, evolution produced such a rapid inflation of complexity and diversity, that it has come to be known as an "explosion". A third point remains to be made and is the subject of this section. Let us consider a thought experiment.

Imagine that we are robots. We are made out of metal, and our brains are composed of large scale integrated circuits made of silicon or some other semi-conductor. Imagine further, that we have no experience of carbon based life. We have never seen it, never heard of it, nor ever contemplated it. Now suppose a robot enters the scene with a flask containing methane, ammonia, hydrogen, water and a few dissolved minerals. This robot asks our academic gathering: "Do you suppose we could build a computer out of this material." The theoreticians in the group would surely say yes, and propose some approaches to the problem. But the engineers in the group would say: "Why bother when silicon is so much better suited to information processing than carbon."

From our organo-centric perspective the robot engineers might seem naive, but in fact I think they are correct. Carbon chemistry is a lousy medium for information processing. Yet the evolutionary process embodies such a powerful drive to generate information processing systems, that it was able to rig up carbon based contraptions for processing information, capable of generating the beauty and complexity of the human mind. What might such a powerful force for information processing do in a medium designed for that purpose in the first place? It is likely to arrive more quickly at sophisticated information process than evolution in carbon chemistry, and would likely achieve comparable functionality with a greater economy of form and process.

11   Harvest Time

The strategy being advocated in this proposal is to let natural selection do most of the work of directing evolution and producing complex software. This software will be "wild", living free in the digital biodiversity reserve. In order to reap the rewards, and create useful applications, we will need to domesticate some of the wild digital organisms, much as our ancestors began domesticating the ancestors of dogs and corn thousands of years ago.

The process must begin with observation. Digital naturalists must explore the digital jungle, observing and publishing on the natural history, ecology, evolution, behavior, physiology, morphology, and other aspects of the biology of the life forms of the digital ecosystem. Much of this work will be academic, like the work of modern day tropical biologists exploring our organic jungles (which I have been doing for twenty years).

However, occasionally, these digital biologists will spot an interesting information process for which they see an application. At this point, some individuals will be captured and brought into laboratories for closer study, and farms for breeding. Sometimes, breeding may be used in combination with genetic engineering (insertion of hand written code, or code transferred from other digital organisms). The objective will be to enhance the performance of the process for which there is an application, while diminishing unruly wild behavior. Some digital organisms will domesticate better than others, as is true for organic organisms (alligators don't domesticate, yet we can still ranch them for their hides).

Once a digital organism has been bred and/or genetically engineered to the point that it is ready to function as an application for end users, they will probably need to be neutered to prevent them from proliferating inappropriately. Also, they will be used in environments free from the mutations that will be imposed on the code living in the reserve. By controlling reproduction and preventing mutation, their evolution will be prevented at the site of the end user. Also the non-replicating interpreted virtual code, might be translated into code that could execute directly on host machines in order to speed their operation.

The organisms living in the biodiversity reserve will essentially be in the public domain. Anyone willing to make the effort can observe them and attempt to domesticate them. However the process of observation, domestication and genetic engineering of digital organisms will require the development of much new technology. This is where private enterprise can get involved. The captured, domesticated, engineered and neutered software that is delivered to the end user will be a salable product, with the profits going to the enterprise that made the efforts to bring the software from the digital reserve to the market.

It seems obvious that organisms evolving in the network-based biodiversity reserve will develop adaptations for effective navigation of the net. This suggests that the most obvious realm of application for these organisms would be as autonomous network agents. It would be much less likely that this kind of evolution could generate software for control of robots, or voice or image recognition, since network based organisms would not normally be exposed to the relevant information flows. Yet at this point we surely can not conceive of where evolution in the digital domain will lead, so we must remain observant, imaginative in or interpretations of their capabilities, and open to new application possibilities.

12   Commitment

Those who wish to support the digital biodiversity reserve by contributing spare CPU cycles should be prepared to make a long-term commitment. Nobody knows how long it will take for complex software to evolve in the reserve. However, a few years will likely be enough time to shake down the system and get a sense of the possibilities. If the desired complexity does begin to evolve, then the reserve should become a permanent fixture within the net.

The same problems are faced in the creation of reserves for organic biodiversity. Great effort and financial resources are required just to establish the reserves. However, that is only the first step. The objective of the reserves is to limit the extent to which human activity causes the extinction of other species. The survival or extinction of organic species is a process that is played out over vast expanses of time: thousands or millions of years. This means that if our rain forest reserves should be converted into pastures or housing developments a thousand years from now, they will have failed.

The organic companion proposal [18] is focused on the sustainability issue. The present strategy is to insure the long term survival of the nature reserves by finding ways for the surrounding human populations to derive an economic benefit from the presence of the reserves. In Costa Rica, at present, this can most easily be done through nature tourism. In the future other economic activities may be more appropriate, or perhaps some centuries or millennia in the future, humans will be willing to protect other species without the motivation of self-interest.

Similar concerns apply to the sustainability of the digital reserve. If the Tierra process provides no reward to those who run it on their nodes, they are likely to terminate the process within a few days, weeks, or months. Such a short participation would be meaningless. As an initial hedge against this problem, a tool will be distributed to allow anyone to observe activity at any participating node, from any node. Yet even this may not be enough, as such tools don't tell a lot about what is going on. To really know the interesting details requires greater effort than most contributors of CPU cycles will have time for.

An even more serious problem is that experience with operation of the system will certainly lead to redesign requiring reinstallation. The ideal situation would be to have the reinstallation done by the same people who do the redesign. However, this would be likely to require that the designers of the reserve actually have accounts on the participating nodes. Where the designers don't have accounts, the contributors would have to do the reinstallation themselves, and they would likely tire of the chore.

The willingness of people to support the reserve for the long term is likely to depend initially on the level of faith that people put in the evolutionary process as a potential generator of rewarding digital processes. Eventually, if all goes well, the harvest of some complex and beautiful digital organisms will provide rewards beyond our imaginations, and should replace faith with solid proof and practice.

13   Containment

The Tierra system is a containment facility for digital organisms. Because Tierra implements a virtual computer, one that has never been implemented in hardware, the digital organisms can only execute on the virtual machine. On any real machine, Tierran organisms are nothing but data. They are no more likely to be functional on a real computer than a program that is executable on a Mac is likely to run on an IBM PC, or that the data in a spread sheet is likely to replicate itself by executing on a machine.

Similarly, the network version of Tierra will create a virtual sub-net, within which the digital organisms will be able to move freely. However, the Tierran digital organisms will not access the real net directly. All communication between nodes will be mediated by the simulation software which does not evolve. When Tierran organisms execute a virtual machine instruction that results in communication across the net, that instruction will be interpreted by the simulation software running on the real machine. The simulation software will pass the appropriate information to a Tierra installation on another machine, through established socket based communication channels. These socket communication channels will only exist between Tierra installations at participating nodes. The digital organisms will not be able to sense the presence of real machines or the real net, nor will they have any way of accessing them.

To further understand the nature of the system, consider a comparison between the Tierra program and the mail program. The mail program is installed at every node on the net and can send data to any other node on the net. The data passing between mail programs is generated by processes that are completely out of control: humans. Humans are beyond control, and sometimes actually malicious, yet the messages that they send through the mail program do not cause problems on the net because they are just data. The same is true of the Tierra program. While the processes that generate the messages passing between Tierra installations are wild digital organisms, the messages are harmless data as they pass through the net. The Tierra program that passes the messages does not evolve, and is as well behaved as the mail program.

A related issue is network load. We do not yet know the level of traffic that would be generated by networked installations of Tierra communicating in the manner described. We will place hard limits on the volume of communication allowed to individual digital organisms in order to prevent mutants from spewing to the net. As we start experimenting with the system, we will monitor the traffic levels to determine if it would have a significant impact on network loads. If the loads are significant, additional measures will need to be taken to limit them. This can be done by charging the organisms for their network access so that they will evolve to minimize their access.

References

[1] P. Barton-Davis, *Independent implementation of the Tierra system*, contact: pauld@cs.washington.edu, unpublished.

[2] R. Brooks, Brooks has created his own Tierra-like system, which he calls Sierra. In his implementation, each machine instruction consists of an opcode and an operand. Successive instructions overlap, such that the operand of one instruction is interpreted as the opcode of the next instruction, contact: brooks@ai.mit.edu, unpublished.

[3] C. Darwin, *On the origin of species by means of natural selection or the preservation of favored races in the struggle for life*, Murray, London, 1859.

[4] J. Dayhoff, 1990, *Neural Network Architectures*, Van Nostrand Reinhold, New York, 1990.

[5] M. de Groot, *Primordial soup, a Tierra-like system that has the additional ability to spawn self-reproducing organisms from a sterile soup*, contact: marc@kg6kf.ampr.org, marc@toad.com, marc@remarque.berkeley.edu, unpublished.

[6] L. Feferman, *Simple rules... complex behavior* [video], Santa Fe Institute, Santa Fe, New Mexico, contact: fef@santafe.edu, 1992.

[7] S. J. Gould, *Wonderful life*, W. W. Norton & Company, Inc., 1989.

[8] J. Hertz, A. Krogh, and R. G. Palmer, *Introduction to the theory of neural computation*, Addison-Wesley Publishing Co., Redwood City, CA, 1991.

[9] C. C. Maley, *A model of early evolution in two dimensions*, Masters of Science thesis, Zoology, New College, Oxford University, contact: cmaley@oxford.ac.uk, 1993

[10] C. Mead, *Analog VLSI and neural systems*, Addison-Wesley Publishing Co., Redwood City, CA, 1993.

[11] S. C. Morris, *Burgess shale faunas and the Cambrian explosion*, Science, 246 (1989), pp. 339–346.

[12] T. S. Ray, *An approach to the synthesis of life*, in Artificial Life II, Santa Fe Institute Studies in the Sciences of Complexity, Vol. X, Addison-Wesley Publishing Co., Redwood City, CA, (1991), pp. 371–408.

[13] ——, *Population dynamics of digital organisms*, in Artificial Life II Video Proceedings, Addison Wesley Publishing Co., Redwood City, CA, 1991.

[14] ——, *Is it alive, or is it GA?*, in Proceedings of the 1991 International Conference on Genetic Algorithms, Morgan Kaufmann, San Mateo, CA, (1991), pp. 527–534.

[15] ——, *Evolution and optimization of digital organisms*, in Scientific Excellence in Supercomputing: The IBM 1990 Contest Prize Papers, The Baldwin Press, Athens, GA, 30602, The University of Georgia, (1991), pp. 489–531.

[16] ——, *Tierra.doc*, Documentation for the Tierra Simulator V4.0, Virtual Life, Newark, DE, 1992. The full source code and documentation for the Tierra program is available by anonymous ftp at: tierra.slhs.udel.edu [128.175.41.34] and life.slhs.udel.edu [128.175.41.33], or by contacting the author.

[17] ——, *An evolutionary approach to synthetic biology: Zen and the art of creating life*, Artificial Life, 1(1/2) (1994), pp. 195–226.

[18] ——, *A proposal to consolidate and stabilize the rain forest reserves of the Sarapiquí region of Costa Rica*, available by anonymous ftp: tierra.slhs.udel.edu [128.175.41.34] and life.slhs.udel.edu [128.175.41.33] as tierra/doc/reserves.tex, 1994.

[19] ——, *Evolution and complexity*, in Complexity: Metaphors, Models, and Reality, Addison-Wesley Publishing Co., Redwood City, CA, (1994), pp. 161–173.

[20] ——, *Evolution, complexity, entropy, and artificial reality*, Physica D 75: 239–263.

[21] K. Thearling, and T. S. Ray, *Evolving multi-cellular artificial life*, Artificial Life IV conference proceedings, In press.

Chapter 5
Information Representation and Self-Organization of the Primary Visual Cortex

Shigeru Tanaka*

Abstract

We often say, "the brain processes information." But this statement is completely meaningless and will not give us any insight to brain function, unless we know what the information stands for. So, we need to know what conveys the information and what is the substrate for the representation of that information. To characterize the visual information, it is convenient to see what visual cortical neurons respond to. The visual stimulus which induces firing of neurons optimally is called the receptive field. Therefore, the receptive field characterizes the visual information processed by individual neurons. This means that what information is processed in the visual cortex is equivalent to which receptive fields are possessed by individual neurons. The receptive field is determined by the neural connectivity from one area to another along the visual pathway in the brain. Consequently, we need to know the connectivity in the visual pathway. It is known that specific neural connections are self-organized depending on the neural activity during development. This indicates that we have to understand mechanisms for synaptic specification processes in order to obtain visual information representation as cortical maps. This is the reason I have focused on the modeling of self-organization of synaptic connections. Major questions discussed in this paper are as follows: (1) How are receptive fields and cortical maps self-organized? (2) What role does visual experience play during cortical development? (3) What is the topological relationship between receptive field profiles and cortical map singularities?

*Exploratory Research Laboratory, Fundamental Research Laboratories, NEC, 34 Miyukigaoka, Tsukuba, Ibaraki 305, Japan and Laboratory for Neural Networks, Frontier Research Program, The Institute of Physical and Chemical Research (RIKEN), 2-1 Hirosawa, Wako, Saitama 351-01, Japan. Present address: Laboratory for Neural Modeling, Frontier Research Program, The Institute of Physical and Chemical Research (RIKEN), 2-1 Hirosawa, Wako, Saitama 351-01, Japan

1   Introduction

Each neuron of the mammalian primary visual cortex responds optimally to a particular pattern of light stimulation within a restricted region of the visual field, which is termed its receptive field (RF). RFs can be specified by several parameters such as ocular dominance, optimal orientation of light or dark bar stimuli, and positions of RF centers. Since Hubel and Wiesel's experiments (1962, 1968), it has been well known that modular structures, with respect to some of these parameters, exist in the visual cortex. Ocular dominance columns (ODCs), center-type patches (CTPs) and orientation preference maps (OPMs) are representative modular structures. These structures are thought to serve as neural substrates for visual information representation.

Since the pioneering work by von der Malsburg (1973), the understanding of mechanisms of column formation has been one of the major targets of theoretical neuroscience. Recently, several mathematical models [11, 33] reproduced surprisingly realistic columnar patterns based on a principle of continuous mapping of the self-organizing feature map [23]. In these studies, the *a priori* existence of the ocular dominance, optimal orientation and positions of RF centers were assumed, without discussing RF formation itself. On the contrary, Linsker showed the spontaneous emergence of oriented RFs from presynaptic concentric RFs in hierarchical linear networks, and then demonstrated that an OPM can be reproduced in the successive layer using only even-symmetric oriented RFs [26]. However, to be able to understand underlying biological mechanisms for column formation, we first need to discuss RF formation within the neuronal layer under consideration, and then extract several parameters from each RF profile to reproduce columnar structure in that layer [32, 31]. This procedure will be followed in this study.

Hebbian learning rules [15], based upon which most self-organization models were built [47, 38, 26, 39, 30], are believed to be mathematical counterparts of mechanisms for synaptic plasticity [9, 12, 22]. These rules state that the co-occurrence of pre- and postsynaptic activities is required for long-term changes in synaptic transmission efficiency. In spite of their similarity - all these models assume some sort of Hebbian rule, they differ in that different constraints have been imposed on the synaptic connection strength.

In the present paper, we first discuss the development of geniculo-cortical projections of animals reared under the binocular deprivation of form vision. The driving force for the orderly map formation is attributed to both cortical interaction among synapses and correlation in activity of cells in the lateral geniculate nucleus (LGN), which are formulated in the Hamiltonian (i.e., the energy function) of the system. The correlation function of neuronal activities is derived from the assumption that afferent inputs from ON- and OFF-center cells compete with each other according to the anti-correlation of firing between them [32, 31], and that there is no correlation between inputs from the left and right eyes because of the lack of visually organized input [32]. The statistical independence in activities between left- and right-eye specific pathways and the anti-correlation of firings between opposite center-type neurons in the LGN give rise to irregular patchy patterns, which resemble ODCs [2] and CTPs observed in the cat visual cortex [14].

Neuronal responses to oriented bar stimuli presented to the retinas are examined in the model visual cortex. Oriented RFs with separate ON and OFF subfields are shown to emerge from the competition between the geniculate afferent inputs from ON- and OFF-center cells with concentric RFs. This shows that visual cortical neurons can become oriented even if animals are reared without form vision [32]. Analysis of simulated RFs clarifies that ON and OFF subfields are composed of direct excitatory inputs from ON- and OFF-center geniculate cells, respectively [32]. This is consistent with Hubel and Wiesel's idea of the composition of simple-cell RFs [18], which has recently been demonstrated by recording from geniculate afferent inputs [8]. The formation of oriented RFs is shown to require the disruption of the precise topographic correspondence between the visual space and the cortical plane [32].

Although the thermodynamic model demonstrates that experimentally observed maps can be generated according to correlation properties in spontaneous firing of LGN cells, it is found that there are some serious discrepancies between simulated results and experimental observations in animals reared under visually normal environments [41]. That is, the RFs of binocular cells are dissimilar, and the tuning of orientation preferences of individual cells is much broader than those experimentally observed. These discrepancies suggest the importance of visual experience during development, which have not been taken into account in the model studied so far. It is also suggested that afferent inputs are self-organized under synergetic effects of visual experience and modifiable intracortical connections.

Furthermore, it is demonstrated that the homotopy theory can explain arrangements of RFs of simple cells around orientation centers, i.e., point singularities in the OPM. The optimal orientation and phase of the RFs can be mapped to the Klein bottle, which is a non-orientable, two-dimensional manifold. Two types of orientation centers have been observed according to clockwise or counterclockwise rotation in optimal orientation. The present topological analysis leads to further classification of these centers whether the RFs of cells in the vicinity of the points are of an ON-center OFF-flank or

OFF-center ON-flank type. In addition, the analysis suggests the existence of a third type of point singularity with respect to the optimal phase.

2 Mathematical Framework for the Self-Organization of Afferent Inputs

Generally, mathematical models which describe the activity-dependent self-organization of afferent inputs require some constraints on synaptic connection strength as well as Hebbian learning rules [47, 38, 26, 39, 30]. The constraints are needed to avoid the divergence of synaptic connection strengths, whereas the Hebbian rules play an important role in generating ordered arrangements of synaptic connections.

In my previous research [40], I postulated a hypothesis involving the competition among synapses for trophic factors. Synapses were assumed to be modified and maintained by trophic factors that might be secreted from target neurons and glial cells. By combining the effects of these factors with a local Hebbian rule, a dynamical equation for synaptic connections was obtained. Close examination of steady-state solutions to this equation showed that the competition among synapses for the limited amount of the factor from the target cells leads to a strong winner-take-all mechanism, which enables us to express the solutions by Potts spin variables [48]. Thereby, the Hamiltonian for the self-organization of the system is clearly described. The degree of synaptic modifiability was assumed to be controlled by the amount of the factor secreted from the glial cells. This effect has been related to the effective temperature in the light of thermodynamics.

As will be seen later, afferent arborization is unstable when there is strong competition among synaptic terminals due to anti-correlation in activity between presynaptic ON- and OFF-center neurons. As a consequence of the Hebbian rule, synaptic terminals originating in some presynaptic cells are often completely eliminated while other presynaptic cells innervate large target areas. To avoid this instability of synaptic terminal arborization, a constraint is required on the number of afferent terminals per presynaptic cell. In this study, a restriction term is introduced in the Hamiltonian, as in the cost function of the artificial neural networks applied to combinatorial optimization problems [17]. This restriction term can be interpreted as the competition among synapses for the limited amount of synaptic maintenance factors, which might be produced at the presynaptic cell bodies.

Here, I show the resulting Hamiltonian H (Appendix A) which completely determines the behavior of the system,

$$H = -\sum_{j,j'} \sum_{\substack{k \in B_j, \mu_1, \mu_2 \\ k' \in B_j, \mu_1', \mu_2'}} V_{j;j'}^{post} \Gamma_{k,\mu_1,\mu_2;k',\mu_1',\mu_2'}^{pre} \sigma_{j,k,\mu_1,\mu_2} \sigma_{j,k',\mu_1',\mu_2'}$$

(1) $$-\sum_j \sum_{k \in B_j, \mu_1, \mu_2} \phi_{k,\mu_1,\mu_2} \sigma_{j,k,\mu_1,\mu_2} + \frac{c}{2} \sum_{k,\mu_1,\mu_2} \left(\sum_j \sigma_{j,k,\mu_1,\mu_2} - \bar{n} \right)^2$$

The first term on the right hand side is given by the synaptic interaction function $V_{j;j'}^{post}$ determined by lateral connections, the presynaptic correlation function of firings between a pair of neurons $\Gamma_{k,\mu_1\mu_2;k',\mu_1'\mu_2'}^{pre}$ and the distribution of afferent synaptic terminals $\{\sigma_{j,k,\mu_1\mu_2}\}$. Subscripts j and k indicate the position of synaptic terminals and the position of presynaptic cell bodies, respectively. Subscripts μ_1 and μ_2 stand for the ocularity and center type of presynaptic cells. When the presynaptic cell receives specific input from the left eye $\mu_1 = +1$, and when the cell receives specific input from the right eye $\mu_1 = -1$. Likewise, when the presynaptic cell is of the ON-center type $\mu_2 = +1$ and otherwise, $\mu_2 = -1$.

The set of presynaptic neurons which can send synaptic connections to position j in the postsynaptic layer are given by B_j. The probability of existence of terminals of afferent inputs from the presynaptic neuron at position k to synaptic position j is assumed to depend on the distance between k and the topographically corresponding position K_j. This probability is given by

(2) $$P_{k;j} = \exp\left(-\frac{d_{k;K_j}^2}{2\lambda_{Arb}^2} \right)$$

where λ_{Arb} determines the extent of possible afferent arborization.

The second term on the right-hand side of Eq. (1) is a bias term in which $\phi_{k,\mu_1\mu_2}$ represents afferent inputs and/or strengths of transmitted activities. If animals are reared under monocular deprivation, then $\phi_{k,\mu_1\mu_2}$ takes different values for $\mu_1 = +1$ and -1 [44, 45]. However, we are currently interested in cases of uniform afferent inputs and balanced activities passing through the inputs, and hence $\phi_{k,\mu_1\mu_2}$ will be fixed at zero without loss of generality.

The last term of Eq.(1), introduced for the first time in this research, imposes a restriction so that the number of synaptic terminals of a presynaptic neuron $n_{k,\mu_1,\mu_2} = \sum_j \sigma_{j,k,\mu_1,\mu_2}$ tends to be the average number $\bar{n}$.

If the value of the coefficient c is too large, then the system cannot change. On the other hand, if it is too small, then the distribution of the number of synaptic terminals are scattered to a large extent. In this case, some of the presynaptic neurons cannot send connections to the target layer while the remaining presynaptic neurons project their afferent inputs predominantly over the postsynaptic layer, as will be shown later.

2.1   Synaptic Interaction Function

The spatial dependence of the function representing synaptic interaction, which was maintained unchanged during self-organization, was assumed to be short-range-excitatory and long-range-inhibitory [37, 40]. It is given by a difference of Gaussian functions:

$$(3) \qquad V_{j;j'}^{post} = \frac{q_{ex}}{2\pi\lambda_{ex}^2}\exp\left(-\frac{d_{j;j'}^2}{2\lambda_{ex}^2}\right) - \frac{q_{inh}}{2\pi\lambda_{inh}^2}\exp\left(-\frac{d_{j;j'}^2}{2\lambda_{inh}^2}\right).$$

Parameters q_{ex} and q_{inh} represent excitatory and inhibitory interaction strengths, which are given by the integration of each part of the function with respect to position j'. Consequently, the average cortical activity is given by $q_{ex} - q_{inh}$. Cortical neurons exhibit spontaneous firing which implies that the average membrane potential is larger than the resting level. That is, the average cortical activity $q_{ex} - q_{inh}$ is positive. Therefore, the value of the ratio of q_{inh} to q_{ex}, should be less than 1. Parameters λ_{ex} and λ_{inh} represent excitatory and inhibitory interaction lengths.

Our synaptic interaction function includes the effect of connections through dendritic fields and each afferent terminal connects specifically to the target cells according to the probability determined by the magnitude of dendritic arborization. This formulation is justified by the notion that each cell receives input from all afferents that arborize within its dendritic fields [4].

2.2   Presynaptic Correlation Function

The presynaptic correlation function $\Gamma_{k,\mu_1,\mu_2;k',\mu_1',\mu_2'}^{pre}$ describes the correlation in activity between two neurons in the LGN (representing the presynaptic layer). For simplicity, if we assume that the LGN serves only as a relay nucleus and does not contribute any additional information processing, the presynaptic correlation function can be looked upon as the correlation function defined in the layer of retinal ganglion cells [43]. Thus, we have to discuss the correlation properties of the retinal ganglion cells.

Organized visual input from the environment may be able to cause correlated firings between separated retinal ganglion cells in the same retina, and binocularly cooperated input may be able to cause correlated firings of ganglion cells between the left and right retinas. However, in this study, these correlated firings are omitted since animals are assumed to be reared in the absence of binocular form vision.

Correlation properties measured in the retinal ganglion cells of cats show that neurons of the opposite center types whose RFs are overlapped tend to fire out of phase while neurons of the same center types tend to fire in phase [28]. This indicates that the value of the correlation function should be positive between same center-type presynaptic neurons and negative between the opposite center-type neurons. The spatial profile of the correlation function is given by the convolution of RFs of two retinal ganglion cells. The detailed derivation of the presynaptic correlation function will be described in Appendix B. As a result, it is given by

$$
(4) \qquad \Gamma^{pre}_{k,\mu_1,\mu_2;k',\mu'_1,\mu'_2} = 2\gamma^P \delta_{\mu_1,\mu'_1}\mu_2\mu'_2 \sum_m R^G_{k;m}R^G_{k';m},
$$

where $R^G_{k;m}$ stands for the ON-center type RF of a retinal ganglion cell, and is given by the following DOG (difference of Gaussian) function:

$$
(5) \qquad R^G_{k;m} = \frac{q_c}{2\pi\lambda_c^2}\exp\left(-\frac{d_{k;m}^2}{2\lambda_c^2}\right) - \frac{q_p}{2\pi\lambda_c^2}\exp\left(-\frac{d_{k;m}^2}{2\lambda_p^2}\right).
$$

where the parameters q_c and q_p represent the strengths of the center and periphery of the RF, respectively, λ_c and λ_p represent the corresponding lengths. Note that $q_c < q_p(q_c > q_p)$ means the suppression (facilitation) of retinal ganglion cell's activity in response to uniform light stimulation which covers its RF.

2.3   Receptive Field Profiles

In formulating the RF which describes neuronal responses to visual stimuli, linear response framework is adopted. In this framework, the RF is defined as the fluctuation of neuronal activity in response to fluctuations in stimulus intensity.

$$(6) \qquad R^{VC}_{j,m,\mu_1} = \sum_{j'} \sum_{\mu_2} \sum_{k'} V^{post}_{j;j'} \sigma_{j',k',\mu_1,\mu_2} \mu_2 R^{G}_{k';m}.$$

The meaning of this equation is that the fluctuations in stimulus are propagated through the afferent inputs $\sigma_{j',k',\mu_1,\mu_2}$ and then summed up by the cortical lateral connections and the dendritic fields $V^{post}_{j;j'}$ to produce membrane polarization at a cortical neuron. The binocular RF is given by the simple sum of the two monocular RFs:

$$(7) \qquad R^{VC}_{j,m,B} = R^{VC}_{j,m,+1} + R^{VC}_{j,m,-1}.$$

3   Simulated Results of the Self-Organization of Afferent Inputs

3.1   Method of computer simulation

The visual cortex is modeled by a square plane of 160 x 160 pixels. The LGN is modeled as four square planes of 20 x 20 neurons, which represent neuronal layers composed of the left ON-center, left OFF-center, right ON-center, and right OFF-center cells. The model of the LGN is supported by experimental evidence of laminar segregation in the LGN of the mink and ferret [25, 36].

First of all, a synaptic connection pattern is prepared as a regular topographic projection from the LGN to the visual cortex. The initial pattern of synaptic connections for Monte Carlo computer simulations are obtained by 4×10^5 random exchanges of the positions of randomly selected pairs of adjacent synaptic terminals. In these random exchanges, each synaptic terminal diffuses within the extent allowed by the probability given by Eq. (2).

The main part of the simulation conforms to the Monte Carlo technique [29] in which a synaptic terminal at a randomly selected position is replaced with another terminal according to the value of the probability. It is determined by the energy difference between the states before and after the replacement, as follows:

$$(8) \qquad \text{Prob}(before \rightarrow after) = \frac{1}{1 + \exp[\beta(E^{after} - E^{before})]}.$$

One Monte Carlo step is defined as 160 x 160 repetitions of trials of the

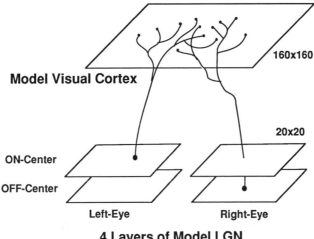

160x160

Model Visual Cortex

20x20

ON-Center

OFF-Center

Left-Eye   Right-Eye

4 Layers of Model LGN

FIG. 1.   *The configuration of afferent inputs from the model LGN to the model visual cortex in the computer simulation. Four types of cells: left ON-center, left OFF-center, right ON-center and right OFF-center cells in the model LGN represented by the square panels send afferent inputs to the dendritic field of the model visual cortex.*

synaptic terminal replacements. When the system reaches equilibrium, in which case the energy takes a constant value, the Monte Carlo simulation ceases.

The values of parameters used in the simulation are as follows: For simplicity, q_{ex} and λ_{inh} were fixed at $q_{ex} = 1$, and $\lambda_{inh} = 1$, and likewise, q_c and λ_p were fixed at $q_c = 1$ and $\lambda_p = 1$. The possible extent of afferent arbor was given by $\lambda_{Arb} = 2.0$. The size of one pixel in the model visual cortex was fixed at 0.08, which leads to 0.32 for the size of one pixel in the four layers of the model LGN. The value of the coefficient c in the restriction term was chosen so that the average value of the restriction is one fourth of the average value of the energy difference during simulation. To see the effects of the restriction, the simulation was also conducted for $c=0.0$. The inverse temperature was fixed at $\beta = 4000$. The values of parameters concerning the synaptic interaction function and the presynaptic correlation function were as follows: $q_{ex} = 1.0, q_{inh} = 0.6, \lambda_{ex} = 0.5, \lambda_{inh} = 1.0, q_c = 1.0, q_p = 0.8, \lambda_c = 0.4,$ and $\lambda_p = 1.0$.

3.2   Effect of Initial Patterns

The initial pattern of afferent synaptic terminals was prepared according to the randomization procedure described above. Afferent terminals were

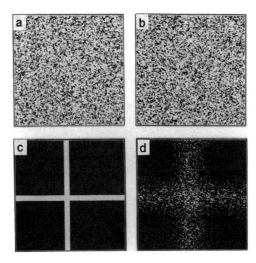

FIG. 2.   *Initial patterns of afferent inputs. Black and white dots in* (a) *indicate the positions of synaptic terminals originating from the presynaptic cells in the left- and right-eye specific layers in the model LGN, irrespective of their center types. Black and white dots in* (b) *indicate the positions of synaptic terminals originating from the ON- and OFF-center layers in the model LGN, irrespective of their ocularities. Black dots in* (d) *represent the positions of synaptic terminals from the cells on the cross-shaped territory in the model LGN shown in* (c).

randomly distributed with respect to ocularity and center type of afferent inputs (Figs. 2a and b). The black dots represent the positions of afferent inputs from the left-eye layer for Fig. 2a and from the ON-center layer for Fig. 2b. The topographic projection is found to be roughly preserved (Figs. 2c and d). This can be seen by the fact that the distribution of afferent inputs from the cross-shaped domain in the model LGN (Fig. 2c) shows a similar pattern (Fig. 2d). Note that distinct patterns emerge from the same initial pattern for independent sessions of Monte Carlo simulation (even for the same values of parameters involved in the synaptic interaction function and the presynaptic correlation function).

3.3   Effect of Restriction Term

Figures 3(a) and (b), and Figs. 3(c) and (d) depict simulated results for different values of the restriction coefficients, $c \neq 0$ and $c=0$, respectively. Patchy patterns of afferent input terminals for the ocularity and the center type were obtained for both cases (Figs. 3(a) and (c)). Patch sizes of the ODC and CTP patterns shown in Fig. 3(c) were notably larger than those of the patterns shown in Fig. 3(a), however.

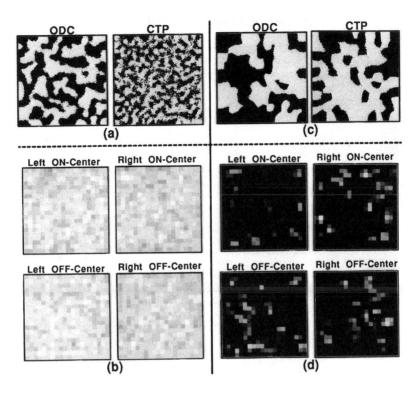

FIG. 3. *Simulated ODC and CTP patterns are shown for $c \neq 0$ in* (a) *and for $c = 0$ in* (c). *The number of synaptic terminals of individual cells in the model LGN normalized by the maximum number for the combination of the ocularity and center type are displayed by the gray level for $c \neq 0$ in* (b) *and for $c = 0$ in* (d).

In Figs. 3(b) and (d), the gray level of each pixel represents the number of afferent input terminals possessed by a model LGN neuron normalized by the maximum number of LGN neurons. For a finite value of c, the fluctuation in the number of afferent inputs possessed by each LGN neuron is very small, because the brightness of the pixels are almost constant (Fig. 3(b)). On the other hand, for $c=0$, the number of afferent terminals of individual presynaptic cells deviate widely from the averaged value $\bar{n} = 16$ (Fig. 3d) since the fluctuation in brightness of the pixels is large (Fig. 3(d)). If such an extremely nonuniform distribution of afferent terminals is realized, visual cortical neurons cannot detect a whole image presented to the retinas since many retinal ganglion cells do not send synaptic inputs to the visual cortex. This may not be the case in reality. The difficulty is that although we need a non-vanishing value for the restriction coefficient, too strong a restriction leads to very slow updating of synaptic connections during the simulation. Consequently, we should choose moderate values for the restriction coefficient c.

3.4   Ocular Dominance Columns and Center-Type Patches

It was found that simulated patterns of ODCs tends to correlate with the ratio of λ_{ex} to λ_{inh}, i.e., the shape of the synaptic interaction function. When the value of $\lambda_{ex}/\lambda_{inh}$ decreases, the ODC period decreases. However, the CTP period does not seem to depend on this value. If the parameter $\lambda_{ex}/\lambda_{inh}$ vanishes, the ODC period goes to infinity (not shown). Therefore, it turns out that the segregation of ODCs is mainly promoted by the synaptic interaction function. In the author's previously proposed Ising spin model [42, 39, 43, 44, 45] as well as in Swindale's model (1980) for ODC formation, the periodicity was reported to be determined by parameters involved in the synaptic interaction function. In these models, the presynaptic correlation function was regarded as a constant-valued function. Consequently, mode selection in ODC formation in the present model seems to obey the same mechanism as in the previous simple models.

However, segregated patterns of ODCs qualitatively differ, in that the simple models reproduce straight stripe ODC patterns whereas the present model gives rise to irregular patchy patterns. The difference in simulated ODC patterns may be attributed to the involvement in ON- and OFF-center inputs, since ON- and OFF-center inputs are taken into account in this study but not in the previous one [39, 44, 45].

In experiments, ODC patterns were found to be straight stripes in monkeys [20] and irregular beaded patches in cats [2]. Since the competition between ON- and OFF-center inputs produced the irregular ODCs shown in Fig. 2a, while the absence of the competition produced straight stripe patterns [43, 44, 45], this indicates that ON- and OFF-center pathways interact with each other in the input layer of the primary visual cortex of cats while they do not in monkeys. Furthermore, this implies that for monkeys, ON- and OFF-center afferent terminals may segregate into different sub-layers within a recipient layer of parvocellular geniculate inputs (layer $4C\beta$) so that these two types of inputs cannot interact with each other.

3.5   Neuronal Responses to Oriented Bar Stimuli

The RFs of simple cells are composed of ON and OFF subfields in which the exposure to light stimuli facilitates and suppresses the neuronal activity. The RFs consist of alternate regions of positive and negative response. These regions are elliptical and aligned parallel to the axis of preferred orientation. Therefore, the cell responses are maximal with optimally oriented gratings located at proper positions within their RFs.

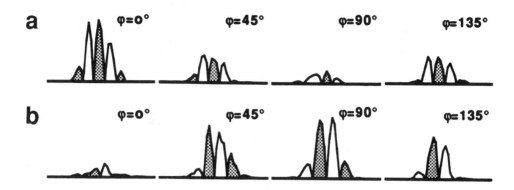

FIG. 4.   *Response curves of three representative simulated cortical cells for four stimulus orientations (0°, 45°, 90°, and 125°). The open and hatched areas represent the strength of neuronal activity in response to light and dark bar stimuli, respectively. The stimuli were assumed to be presented to both eyes at the same time.*

Binocular responses of representative model cortical neurons to oriented bar stimuli for four orientations are shown in Fig. 4. This figure depicts the dependence of neuronal response strength on the position of the bar along the axis perpendicular to the bar orientation. The height of the response curves represents firing rate induced by bar stimuli, where responses to light and dark stimuli are shown by open and hatched areas, respectively. Therefore, those areas with open and hatched responses correspond to ON and OFF subfields. The shape and amplitude of the response curves change for different bar orientations. Oscillatory curves for the responses can be seen clearly for the bar orientation that induces the strongest responses, that is, the optimal orientation.

3.6   Two-Dimensional Structure of Receptive Fields

Having seen the separation of ON and OFF subfields characteristic of simple cells in the model cortical neurons above, two-dimensional arrangements of ON and OFF subfields according to Eqs. (5) and (6) are shown in Fig. 5. A large majority of these RFs are oriented (Figs. 5a and b), even though the simulation assumed isotropic intracortical connections as well as concentric RFs of presynaptic cells. These oriented RFs can be fitted by the Gabor function at position $\vec{x}$ in the visual space measured from its center position

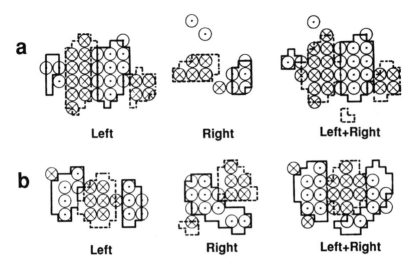

FIG. 5.   *Two-dimensional RF profiles of four representative cortical cells and their compositions of afferent inputs. The left, middle and right columns illustrate left-eye monocular, right-eye monocular and binocular RFs. The cortical ON and OFF subfields are surrounded by the solid and dotted lines, respectively. Cell **a** exhibits left-eye dominance in response to stimuli. Cell **b** is binocularly responsive; the optimal orientation for left-eye stimulation differs from that for right-eye stimulation but the binocular optimal orientation is close to the left-eye orientation since the ocular dominance is slightly shifted to the left eye. Presynaptic RF centers are plotted with circles containing a dot for ON-center cells and circles containing a cross for OFF-center cells. It is found that the presynaptic ON- and OFF-center RFs overlap with the ON and OFF subfields of the model cortical cells.*

as follows: $R(\vec{x}) = A\exp\left(-\frac{\vec{x}^2}{2\sigma^2}\right)\cos[2\pi f \ \vec{e}\ (\theta)\cdot\ \vec{x}\ -\phi]$, where θ and ϕ stand for the optimal orientation and the optimal phase, and A, σ, f and $\vec{e}$ represent the normalization factor of the RF, width of the RF, spatial frequency and unit vector vertical to the orientation θ respectively. This is also consistent with the fact that physiologically observed simple cells are well modeled by the same function [27, 10]. It should be noted that simple-cell RF profiles are specified by the optimal orientation and phase. On the other hand, a small minority were found to be unoriented or to possess more complicated RFs. Generally, profiles of monocular RFs of binocularly responsive neurons differ for left and right monocular vision (Fig. 5b).

Computer simulations were conducted for different values of $\lambda_{ex}/\lambda_{inh}$ to examine the dependence of cortical RF profiles on presynaptic RF profiles. For large values of $\lambda_{ex}/\lambda_{inh}$, cortical RFs tend to be exclusively ON or OFF responsive types (E-ON or E-OFF types). On the other hand, for small values of the ratio, the RFs are likely to have separate ON and OFF subfields. This indicates that the ratio in diameter of the center subfield to the surround subfield for the LGN cells determines the types of the cortical RFs.

As pointed out above, the size of CTPs correlates with the areas of the ON and OFF subfields. When the patch size is large, the area of each subfield is large, and hence E-ON (or E-OFF) RFs tend to emerge.

Cortical neurons of normally reared animals are known to have the same orientation preference in the two eyes, when the RFs in each eye are examined by monocular stimulation [18]. However, the simulation showed that optimal orientations of individual neurons in the two eyes seem to be independent. This can be attributed to the absence of binocular organized inputs. Even though oriented RFs may be formed by the spontaneous symmetry breaking mechanism, as we have seen, binocular form vision during development plays an important role for the agreement of left and right monocular orientation preferences for binocular cells.

I have also investigated how ON and OFF responsive subfields in the cortical RFs are composed of inputs from the presynaptic ON- and OFF-center neurons. Figure 5 also shows arrangements of ON- and OFF-center subfields of the model LGN neurons, which directly send their axons in the vicinity of the cortical neurons under consideration. In Fig. 5, it can be seen that ON- and OFF-center subfields of LGN neurons overlap with the ON and OFF subfields of cortical neurons, respectively. Furthermore, the arrangements of the presynaptic RF centers were elongated, having an inclination parallel to the optimal orientation of the cortical neurons (Figs. 5a and b). E-ON and E-OFF neuron's RFs were composed of afferent inputs from the presynaptic neurons of the same center types (Figs. 5c). Even when the cortical lateral inhibition and surround part of the presynaptic RF were abolished, simulated cortical RFs had the same arrangements of ON and OFF subfields. Therefore the RF profiles are mainly determined by afferent excitatory inputs.

The fact that each subfield is composed of presynaptic RFs of the same center type strongly supports the mechanism of RF formation in simple cells through the linear alignment of ON- and OFF-center presynaptic RFs along the lengths of ON and OFF subfields. This theoretical result is consistent with the experimental evidence given by recordings from cortical neurons and adjacent geniculate afferents following suppression of cortical neuron's activity by GABA antagonistic chemicals in the ferret visual cortex [8]. These theoretical and experimental data justify Hubel and Wiesel's hypothetical mechanism for the composition of cortical RFs [18].

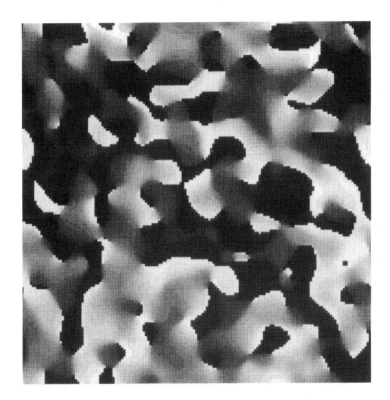

FIG. 6. *Orientation preference map. Horizontal arrangements of optimal orientation obtained from our computer simulation. The optimal orientations of model cortical neurons are represented by six gray levels for visualization, although they change continuously in the model visual cortex. The simulated orientations are regularly arranged except for singularity points. Orientation centers are located at positions where all the optimal orientations converge.*

3.7   Orientation Preference Map

The simulation also reproduced an orderly map of optimal orientations that are arranged continuously almost everywhere along the cortical surface, and this map contains point singularities, i.e., orientation centers [5, 3], at which all orientations from 0° to 180° are represented as a pinwheel-like structure. In Fig. 6, optimal orientations from 0° to 180° are indicated by the gray levels. Therefore, the orientation centers are the points where all gray levels converge.

We have reported that the optimal orientation tends to remain unchanged in the direction across the borders of CTPs and that the optimal phase tends to remain unchanged along the borders of the patches [32]. These spatial relationship of optimal orientation and phase to CTPs indicate that the axis of constant optimal orientation is locally at right angle to the axis of constant optimal phase. This implies that we can define a relevant hypercolumn in which optimal orientations and phases are represented, by analogy to the original hypercolumn for orientations and ocularities [19]. If we assume that any visual pattern should be represented by a set of activities of simple cells, our hypercolumn can serve as the functional basis for representing visual information since it contains a complete set of orientations and phases.

3.8   Topographic Arrangements

When neurons were sampled at the same interval along straight lines in the model visual cortex, the traces of the RF centers in the visual space are shown in Fig. 7. The RF center was defined as the center of mass of presynaptic cells which connect to the cortical cell. This definition is justified by the fact that cortical RFs were determined mainly by excitatory afferent inputs to the cells, as demonstrated in Fig. 5. Figure 7 shows that the trace of RF centers travels back and forth, but the center positions shift, on average, only in one direction. These topographical properties are consistent with experimental observations [1]. The center positions of binocular RFs change smoothly but those of dominant monocular RFs jump discontinuously when the cells change their ocular dominance across ODC borders.

In order to examine overall topography in afferent projections, topographic nets were depicted in Fig. 8. These nets were made by horizontal and vertical traces of RF centers of the cells at vertices on a fictitious square lattice in the model cortex. The monocular topographic nets have holes (Figs. 8a and b). These holes emerge due to the fact that many cortical cells are monocularly responsive. These broken topographic nets show that self-organization does not necessarily lead to continuous topology-preserving maps. The holes as seen in monocular topographic nets vanish in the binocular net, though many wrinkles remain (Fig. 8c). Computer simulations without competition between ON- and OFF-center inputs produced regular topographic maps (not shown). Consequently, the folds and wrinkles in the binocular topographic nets may be due to the competition between ON- and OFF-center afferent inputs. In other words, the emergence of oriented RFs may require the disruption of topography, as pointed out in our previous paper [32]. Comparison of these monocular nets (Figs. 8a and b) with the binocular one (Fig. 8c) clearly indicates that binocular vision compensates for the disruption of monocular topographies. Figures 8c-d illustrate that topographic order depends on the sampling interval of model cortical neurons. It is likely that nets become less folded as the sampling interval becomes larger. Therefore, the local topography is not necessarily preserved,

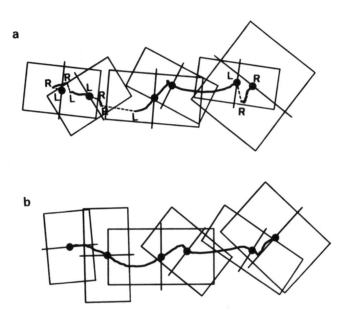

FIG. 7.   *Traces of the simulated cortical RF centers of cells sampled with a regular interval along a line in the model cortex.   Trace* **a** *shows the centers of dominant eye RFs and* **b** *shows the centers of binocular RFs.   The rectangles represent the size of the RFs and the line segments in the middle of the rectangles indicate their optimal orientations.   The dotted lines connect RF centers with opposite ocular dominances when the ocular dominance is reversed across the ODC borders.*

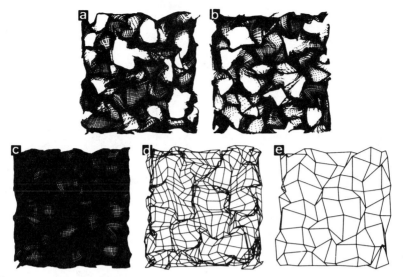

FIG. 8.   *Topographic nets. The vertices in these nets defined in the visual field represent the positions of RF centers for neurons periodically arranged on the cortical plane. The RF centers of cortical cells were determined by the centers of mass of presynaptic cells which connect in the vicinity of the cortical cells.* **a, b** *and* **c** *are the left-eye monocular, right-eye monocular and binocular precise nets, respectively.* **d** *and* **e** *are coarse nets with different intervals of cortical cells.*

even though the global topography. Taken together, synaptic connections are self-organized, so that cortical cells acquire orientation preference with the consequence that topography is wrinkled at precise scales.

4   Effects of Visual Experience

4.1   Discrepancies between simulated results and experimental observations

Tuning curves for two representative oriented cells are shown in Fig. 9 for left-monocular, right-monocular, and binocular responses. Generally, the orientation tuning for binocular RFs is found to be sharper than that for monocular ones. As seen from these curves, the widths of half maxima (about 90°) are larger than the observed widths (about 50° or less) [34]. The tuning width could not be narrowed even when the simulation for the self-organization was extended. Therefore, the broad tuning in simulated results is intrinsic to the model. In order to increase orientation tuning, other factors not considered here, are required.

Optimal orientations for monocular stimulation of cells along a line on

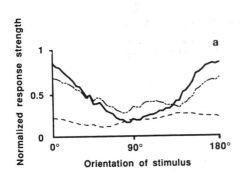
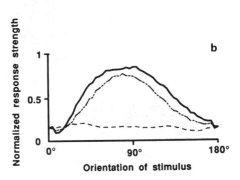

FIG. 9.   *Orientation tuning curves for two representative simulated cortical cells with different optimal orientations. The solid, chained and dashed curves show the activity in response to binocular, left-eye monocular and right-eye monocular oriented bar stimuli. In* **b**, *the left-eye monocular response exhibits orientation selectivity, while the right-eye monocular response shows no orientation selectivity. Response curves* **a** *and* **b** *were taken from the simulated cells shown in Figs. 3**a** and **b**, respectively.*

the model cortex were examined (not shown). They were found to be continuously arranged along the cortex except at the borders of ODCs. These discontinuities in orientation imply that binocular cells, which tend to appear along the ODC borders, have different optimal orientations in the two eyes. As shown in Fig. 10, the histogram of interocular difference in optimal orientation for binocular cells possess a uniform distribution. This also indicates that optimal orientations in the left eye are statistically independent of those in the right eye, as pointed out before. Since only spontaneous firing was assumed in the present model, there is no driving force constraining optimal orientations in the two eyes to agree with each other.

4.2   Requirement of selective learning

These discrepancies are reasonable, because no mechanism for enforcing agreement between optimal orientations in the two eyes was included in the model for the absence of form vision. Therefore, visual experience turns out to be indispensable in order to reproduce highly orientation-selective RFs with similar orientations in the two eyes.

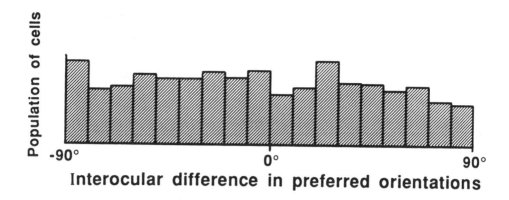

FIG. 10.   *Interocular difference histogram in optimal orientation. The histogram shows a uniform distribution of the difference between optimal orientations in the two eyes. This indicates that optimal orientations in the two eye are statistically independent.*

In order to see how the visual experience affects synaptic changes, let us compare time courses for synaptic changes and for presentations of visual patterns. The former time course is expected to be much longer than the latter (about 100 ms when estimated as the duration of a saccadic eye movement). Even if we assume only the visual experience in the present model for the self-organization of afferent inputs, various kinds of visual patterns are exposed to the retinas during the time course for synaptic changes, and the presynaptic correlation function are statistically averaged to be almost concentric. Therefore, this model does not fundamentally change the model based on spontaneous activities. This means that the effect of visual experience alone cannot reproduce the highly tuned orientation selectivity and the agreement of optimal orientations in the two eyes. Consequently, we need to assume some other effect, in addition to visual experience.

4.3   Involvement of long-range horizontal collaterals

One possible idea is that a template supervises the maturation of the OPM and the agreement of optimal orientations in the two eyes. However, it is hard to assume that the template exists in the visual cortex prior to the formation of OPMs. Therefore, the template should also be formed according to visual experience. In normal rearing conditions, animals see objects in their environments with both eyes. Therefore, it may be that

while lateral excitatory and/or inhibitory connections are matured based
on the binocular OPM, they serve as the template for the formation of
monocular OPMs. That is, lateral connections selectively transmit signals
from the environment according to the neuronal orientation preference.
The orientation selectivity, which is self-organized based on spontaneous
activities before eye opening, may be enhanced by the selective transmission
of signals preferred by particular cortical neurons. I will call such learning
selective learning.

It is well known that in the cerebral cortex, there are intracortical
connections such as long-range horizontal connections in addition to the
afferent inputs. It has been reported that these horizontal connections
link assemblies of neurons during postnatal development [13]. Also,
normal refinement of patchy arbors of the horizontal connections has been
demonstrated to require visual experience [7]. It has been found that the
horizontal connections have a nonlinear transmission of activities depending
on the membrane potential of their recipient cells [16]. This property may
be effective for selective learning. My preliminary computer simulation,
in which this state-dependent signal transmission property is incorporated,
exhibited increased orientation tuning of individual neurons and increased
similarity of monocular optimal orientations in the two eyes compared to
the model cortex [41]. In this case, it was found that the disparity beteween
the left- and right-eye vision maintains the presence of ocular dominance
columns, instead of uncorrelated firing of cells between left- and right-eye
pathways for the model based on spontaneous activities in LGN cells. Thus,
the role of the horizontal connections in a developmental process can be
interpreted as selecting preferentially oriented stimuli as supervising signals.

4.4   Involvement of lateral inhibition

Recently, Komatsu and Iwakiri (1993) have reported that the inhibitory
synaptic transmission to a cortical neuron in developing rats is potentiated
after high-frequency activation of GABAergic inhibitory synapses, while
it is depressed after high-frequency activation of excitatory synapses in
the same neuron. Interestingly, such potentiation and depression of
inhibitory synaptic transmission strongly depends on the age of the rats,
which suggests that the synaptic changes contributes to the postnatal
development of selective responsiveness of visual cortical cells through
visual experience. These observations imply that the co-occurrence of
presynaptic firing and postsynaptic hyperpolarization enhances the synaptic
transmission efficiencies. We may postulate the hypothesis that Inhibitory
lateral connections are changeable according to an anti-Hebbian mechanism.
According to this hypothesis, it is possible that the inhibitory synaptic

interaction function changes to be anisotropic during development. In my preliminary computer simulation (based on a model with an anti-Hebbian rule for lateral inhibition), elongated cortical RFs along the axis of the optimal orientations of the model neurons were obtained. It was also found that individual neurons tend to have similar orientation preferences in the two eyes. The learning of lateral inhibition as well as excitatory long-range horizontal connections may be able to explain the postnatal development of orientation preference in cortical neurons.

To summarize the effect of visual experience in afferent input self-organization: a synergy of visual experience and learning of intracortical connections is indispensable for formation of highly tuned orientation selectivity and related columnar structures observed in the visual cortex of normally reared animals.

5   Topological Analysis of Visual Information Representation

We have seen before that the computer simulation of the self-organization of afferent inputs demonstrated the emergence of orientation centers and pinwheel-like structures in the OPM (Fig. 6). In this section, I will show that such a characteristic feature of the OPM can be explained by the topology of the Klein bottle [6], This topological approach to an understanding of representation of optimal orientation and phase in the visual cortex is expected to provide a hint that will lead to a general understanding of information representation in the cerebral cortex [46].

Although, at first glance, the Klein bottle does not seem to relate to information representation in the visual cortex, it is naturally derived from the RF profile of simple cells, as will be shown in the following. As I pointed out previously, the RF profile of simple cells can be fitted by the Gabor function. Hereafter, two parameters θ and ϕ defined in the rectangular domain: $0° \leq \theta \leq 180°$ and $0° \leq \phi \leq 360°$ will be focused on particularly (Fig. 11a). In this figure, representative RF profiles derived from the Gabor function are illustrated, which should occur along the edges of the domain. The white and black ovals in Fig. 11a show the ON and OFF subfields in the RFs, respectively. It is noted that identical configurations of ON and OFF subfields appear along the opposite edges of the domain, and that these change continuously in the direction indicated by the arrows. Therefore, the directed opposite edges are identical when considering their directions. This domain can be made into a tube by pasting the two identical horizontal edges (Fig. 11b). This tube has directed circles at the two ends. Therefore, in order to paste the two ends together with identical directions, we have to twist the tube into the form of the Klein bottle (Figs. 11c and d).

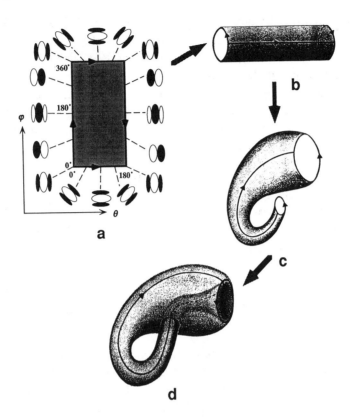

FIG. 11.   *How to make a Klein bottle from symmetry properties of RF profiles.* **a.** *The RF profiles given by the Gabor function are illustrated only at the representative points along the edges of the rectangular domain.* **b.** *Identical RF profiles appear on the opposite edges of the rectangular domain, and they change in the same manner in the direction indicated by the arrows.* **c** *and* **d.** *By pasting the pairs of identical edges together so that their directions coincide, the rectangular domain becomes a Klein bottle. Note that the horizontal and vertical edges of the domain are transformed to closed loops ℓ and n on the Klein bottle.*

Consequently, the horizontal and vertical edges of the rectangular domain are transformed to closed loops ℓ and n on the Klein bottle, respectively.

Since the computer simulation showed that the optimal orientation and phase are continuously represented almost everywhere along the cortex [32], when we move along a given closed loop on the cortical surface, the corresponding trajectory of the orientation and phase should form a closed loop on the Klein bottle. Such closed loops on the Klein bottle are classified into two types according to whether or not they can be reduced by continuous deformation of the loops into points (Fig. 12a and Figs. 12b-d). When a closed loop on the Klein bottle can be shrunk into a point (Fig. 12a), there are no singularities inside of the corresponding cortical closed loop, as shown in Fig. 13a. On the other hand, when closed loops on the Klein bottle cannot be reduced into points (Figs. 12b-d), the corresponding cortical loops contain point singularities (Figs. 13b_1-d). Figures 13b_1 and b_2 correspond to Fig. 12b, but they have different directions of rotations in RFs. Figures 13c_1 and c_2 likewise correspond to Fig. 12c. Figure 13d is a unique case for a loop around the Klein bottle axis shown in Fig. 12d. For the cortical loop in Fig. 13a, contour integration of the gradient of orientation or phase amounts to zero. By contrast, for those loops of Figs. 13b_1 - c_2, the contour integration of the gradient of orientation is ±180° while that of the gradient of phase is zero. For the loop of Fig. 13d, contour integration of the gradient of orientation is zero, while that of the gradient of phase is 360°. Thus, there is one-to-one correspondence between a class of point singularities on the cortical surface and a class of closed loops on the Klein bottle which can be transformed into one another by continuous deformation. If a closed loop turns twice along the Klein bottle axis, it will give rise to an orientation center around which the contour integration of the gradient of orientation amounts to 360°. However, actual maps in the primary visual cortex do not exhibit orientation centers around which the orientation changes by more than 180° [5, 3].

Another interesting feature of the Klein bottle representation of RFs is that a loop over one side of the Klein bottle (ℓ in Fig. 12b) gives rise to ON-center OFF-flank RFs (Figs. 13b_1 and b_2), while a loop over the other side (m in Fig. 12c) gives rise to OFF-center ON-flank RFs (Figs. 13c_1 and c_2), even though the difference in RF types cannot be distinguished in the actual map that represents only the spatial distribution of orientations. From similar topological considerations on the closed loop around the bottle axis (Fig. 12d), it is suggested that such point singularities about the phase can exist between orientation centers.

6   Conclusion

I have formulated the self-organization of neural networks based on the thermodynamics of the Potts spin system [40, 43]. In this formulation, we have two quantities, synaptic connections which are self-organized, and RFs which are determined by the self-organized synaptic connections. These are well-defined biological counterparts from viewpoints of both anatomy and physiology. The introduction of these two quantities enables us to discuss the relationships between the anatomical distribution of afferent synaptic terminals and physiological neuronal properties. In the context of thermodynamics, ordered structures can be interpreted to emerge from initial random patterns by means of spontaneous symmetry breaking mechanisms.

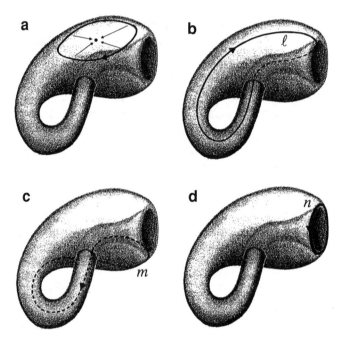

FIG. 12. *Closed loops on the Klein bottle.* **a.** *A closed loop that can be reduced into a point by continuous deformation of the loop. In topology, closed loops can be freely deformed as if they are made from rubber.* **b.** *A closed loop ℓ surrounding the Klein bottle turning once along the top surface of the bottle specified by $\phi = 0°$* **c.** *A closed loop m surrounding the bottle turning once along the bottom surface of the bottle specified by $\phi = 180°$.* **d.** *A closed loop surrounding n the bottle turning once around the bottle axis specified by $\theta = 0°$.*

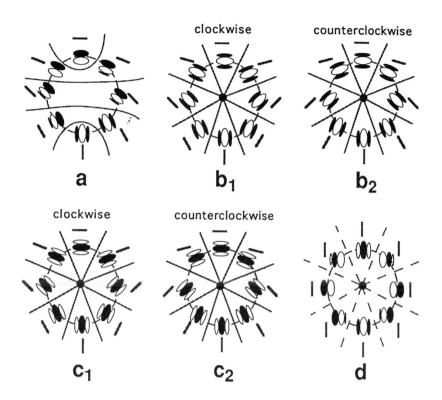

FIG. 13. *Possible configurations of RF profiles and iso-orientation domains in the visual cortex. The orientation of each domain is indicated by the inclination of the short line segments. Point singularities indicated by the dots are contained in* **b** - **c** *but not in* **a**. **a**. *The net increments in angle of the orientation and phase amount to zero for one round-trip along the cortical closed loop, in the case where the corresponding closed loop on the Klein bottle (Fig. 12**a**) can be shrunk into a point.* **b$_1$** *and* **b$_2$**. *When we move counterclockwise along the cortical closed loop, the orientation changes clockwise (**b$_2$**) or counterclockwise (**b$_1$**) by 180° as correlated with a clockwise or counterclockwise rotation along the corresponding loop ℓ on the Klein bottle (Fig. 12**b**).* **c$_1$** *and* **c$_2$**. *When we move counterclockwise along the cortical loop, the orientation changes clockwise (**c$_2$**) or counterclockwise (**c$_1$**) by 180° as correlated with a clockwise or counterclockwise rotation along the corresponding loop m (Fig. 12**c**).* **d**. *When we move along the cortical loop n (Fig. 12**d**), only the phase changes by 360° with the orientation remaining unchanged.*

In the present paper, I applied the theory to the activity-dependent self-organization of geniculate afferent inputs in animals deprived of binocular form vision. A constraint keeping the number of synaptic terminals of individual presynaptic neurons almost constant was included. This constraint proved to be necessary to avoid constructing a disrupted visual field. It is also interpreted as the struggle for existence among synaptic connections for the limited amount per unit time of chemical factors that might be synthesized at each presynaptic neuron.

Irregular patchy patterns that resemble ODCs and CTPs observed in the cat visual cortex were reproduced. These patterns were also shown to emerge due to the absence of correlation in firing between left- and right-eye specific pathways and the anti-correlation in firings between opposite center-type LGN neurons.

Oriented ON and OFF separate subfields emerged from the competition between ON- and OFF-center afferent inputs despite the absence of orientation bias. This shows that visual cortical neurons are able to become oriented even if animals are reared without form vision. Analysis of simulated RFs clearly indicates that ON and OFF subfields are composed of direct excitatory inputs from ON- and OFF-center geniculate cells, respectively. This is consistent with Hubel and Wiesel's idea of the composition of simple-cell RFs. The oriented RFs were formed by the re-arrangement of afferent inputs so that precise topography was broken to some extent.

Disagreements between the simulated results of afferent input self-organization and observations in normally reared animals were clarified. In order to reproduce maps in the normal visual cortex, the need for synergy of visual experience and learning of horizontal connections (which serve as selective learning) was suggested. It was proposed that some combination of long-range horizontal excitations and inhibitions assist the formation of normal cortical maps.

The topological analysis demonstrates that characteristic features of maps with respect to the optimal orientation and phase in the visual cortex can be systematically explained by the of topology the Klein bottle derived from simple-cell RF properties. Similar considerations will apply to RF properties of other types of cells in the primary visual cortex and cells in other cortical areas. I believe that this topological viewpoint will provide us with novel mathematical insights and lead to an understanding of mechanisms of cortical information representation. One possibility is to extend this topological approach to a theory of the "fiber bundle" [35] with the Klein bottle as its "fiber" and the 2-dimensional cortical surface as its "base space". Through this extension, a potentially useful theoretical structure will be introduced to the theory so that we can fruitfully discuss energetically possible point singularities in the visual cortex.

References

[1] K. Albus, *A quantitative study of the projection area of the central and the peripheral visual field in area 17 of the cat, I.*, The precision of the topography. Exp. Brain Res. 24, (1975), pp. 159–179.

[2] P. A. Anderson, J. Olavarria, R. C. Van Sluyters, *The overall pattern of ocular dominance bands in the cat visual cortex.* J. Neurosci. 8, (1988), pp. 2183–2200.

[3] T. Bonhoeffer, A. Grinvald, *Iso-orientation domains in cat visual cortex are arranged in pinwheel-like patterns.*, Nature 353, (1991), pp. 429–431.

[4] G. G. Blasdel, D. Fitzpatrick, *Physiological organization of layer 4 in macaque striate cortex*, J. Neurosci. 4, (1984), pp. 880–895.

[5] G. G. Blasdel, G. Salama, *Voltage-sensitive dyes reveal a modular organization in monkey striate cortex*, Nature 321, (1986), pp. 579–585.

[6] G. E. Bredon, *Topology and Geometry*, Graduate Texts in Mathematics 139. Springer-Verlag, New York Berlin Heidelberg London Paris Tokyo Hong Kong Barcelona Budapest, (1993).

[7] E. M. Callaway and L. C. Katz, *Effects of binocular deprivation on the development of clustered horizontal connections in cat striate cortex*, Proc. Natl. Acad. Sci. USA 88, (1991), pp. 745–749.

[8] B. Chapman, K. R. Zahs, M. P. Stryker, *Relation of cortical cell orientation selectivity to alignment of receptive fields of the geniculocortical afferents that arborize within a single orientation column in ferret visual cortex*, J. Neurosci. 11, (1991), pp. 1347–1358.

[9] G. L. Collingridge and T. V. P. Bliss, *NMDA receptors - their role in long-term potentiation*, Trends in Neurosci. 10, (1987), pp. 288–293.

[10] J. G. Daugman, *Two-dimensional spectral analysis of cortical receptive field profiles*, Vision Research 20, (1980), pp. 847–856.

[11] R. Durbin, G. Mitchison, *A dimension reduction framework for understanding cortical maps*, Nature 343, (1990), pp. 644–647.

[12] E. Frank, *The influence of neuronal activity on patterns of synaptic connections*, Trends in Neurosci 10, (1987), pp. 188–190.

[13] C. D. Gilbert and T. N. Wiesel, *Columnar specificity of intrinsic horizontal and corticocortical connections in cat visual cortex*, J. Neurosci. **9**, (1989), pp. 2432–2442.

[14] J. A. Gordon, E. S. Ruthazer, M. P. Stryker, *Segregation of ON- and OFF-center afferents to cat visual cortex*, Soc. for Neurosci. Absts. 19, (1993), pp. 333.

[15] D. O. Hebb, *The Organization of Behavior.* Wiley, (1949).

[16] J. A. Hirsch, C. D. Gilbert, *Synaptic physiology of horizontal connections in the cat's visual cortex*, J. Neurosci. 11, (1991), pp. 1800–1809.

[17] J. J. Hopfield, D. W. Tank, *"Neural" computation of decisions in optimization problems*, Biol. Cybern. 52, (1985), pp. 141–152.

[18] D. H. Hubel, T. N. Wiesel, *Receptive fields, binocular interaction and functional architecture in the cat's visual cortex*, J. Physiol. 160, (1962), pp. 106–154.

[19] D. H. Hubel, T. N. Wiesel, *Receptive fields and functional architecture of monkey striate cortex*, J. Physiol. 195, (1968), pp. 215–243.

[20] D. H. Hubel, T. N. Wiesel, S. LeVay, *Plasticity of ocular dominance columns in monkey striate cortex* Phil. Trans. R. Soc. Lond. B278, (1977), pp. 377–409.

[21] D. H. Hubel, T. N. Wiesel, *Functional architecture of macaque monkey visual cortex*, Proc. R. Soc. Lond. B198, (1977), pp. 1–59.

[22] A. Kleinschmidt, M. F. Bear and W. Singer, *Blockade of "NMDA" receptors disrupts experience-dependent plasticity of kitten striate cortex*, Science 238, (1987), pp. 355–358.

[23] T. Kohonen, *Self-organized formation of topologically correct feature maps*, Biol. Cybern. 43, (1982), pp. 59–69.

[24] Y. Komatsu, M. Iwakiri, *Long-term modification of inhibitory synaptic transmission in developing visual cortex*, NeuroReport 4, (1993), pp. 907–910.

[25] S. LeVay, S. K. McConnell, *ON and OFF layers in the lateral geniculate nucleus of the mink*, Nature 300, (1982), pp. 561–594.

[26] R. Linsker, *From basic network principles to neural architecture*, Proc. Natl. Acad. Sci. USA 83, (1986), pp. 7508–7512, pp. 8390–8394, pp. 8779–8783.

[27] S. Marcelja, *Mathematical description of the responses of simple cortical cells*, J. Optical. Soc. America 70, (1983), pp. 1297–1300.

[28] D. N. Mastronarde, *Correlated firing of cat retinal ganglion cells. II. Responses of X-and Y-cells to single quantal events*, J. Neurophysiol. 49, (1980), pp. 325–349.

[29] N. Metropolis, A. W. Rosenbluth, M. N. Rosenbluth, A. H. Teller, E. Teller, *Equation of state calculations by fast computing machines*, J. Chem. Phys. 21, (1953), pp. 1087–1092.

[30] K. D. Miller, J. B. Keller, M. P. Stryker, *Ocular dominance column development: Analysis and simulation*, Science 245, (1989), pp. 605–615.

[31] K. D. Miller, *Development of orientation columns via competition between on- and off-center inputs*, NeuroReport 3, (1992), pp. 73–76.

[32] M. Miyashita, S. Tanaka, *A mathematical model for orientation column formation*, NeuroReport 3, (1992), pp. 69–72.

[33] K. Obermayer, H. Ritter, K. Schulten, *A principle for the formation of the spatial structure of cortical maps*, Proc. Natl. Acad. Sci. USA 87, (1990), pp. 8345–8349.

[34] I. Ohzawa, R. D. Freeman, *The binocular organization of simple cells in the cat's visual cortex* J. Neurophysiol. 56, (1986), pp. 221–242.

[35] N. Steenrod, *The topology of fibre bundles*, Princeton, (1972).

[36] M. P. Stryker, K. R. Zahs, *ON and OFF sublaminae in the lateral geniculate nucleus of the ferret*, J. Neurosci. 3, (1983), pp. 1943–1951.

[37] N. V. Swindale, *A model for the formation of ocular dominance stripes*, Proc. R. Soc. Lond. B208, (1980), pp. 243–264.

[38] A. Takeuchi, S-I Amari, *Formation of topographic maps and columnar microstructures in nerve fields*, Biol. Cybern. 35, (1979), pp. 63–72.

[39] S. Tanaka, *Theory of self-organization of cortical maps. In Touretzky DS*, (ed) Advances in neural information processing system 1, Morgan Kaufmann, (1989), pp. 451–458.

[40] S. Tanaka, *Theory of self-organization of cortical maps: mathematical framework*, Neural Networks 3 (1990), pp. 625–640.

[41] S. Tanaka, *A scenario of the postnatal development of columnar organization in striate cortex*, Soc. Neurosci. Absts. 19, (1993), p. 893.

[42] S. Tanaka, *Theory of self-organization of cortical maps*, In The proceeding of SICE '88, ESS2-5, (1988), pp. 1069–1072

[43] S. Tanaka, *Experience-dependent self-organization of biological neural networks*, NEC Research and Development No. 98, (1990), pp. 1–14.

[44] S. Tanaka, *Theory of ocular dominance column formation: Mathematical basis and computer simulation*, Biol. Cybern. 64:, (1991), pp. 263–272.

[45] S. Tanaka, *Phase transition theory for abnormal ocular dominance column formation*, Biol. Cybern. 65, (1991), pp. 91–98.

[46] S. Tanaka, *Topological analysis of point singularities in stimulus preference maps of the primary visual cortex*, Royal Society Proceedings B, (in press).

[47] C. von der Malsburg, *Self-organization of orientation selective cells in the striate cortex*, Kybernetik 14 (1973), pp. 85–100.

[48] F. Y.Wu, *The Potts model*, Rev. Mod. Phys. 54, (1982), pp. 235–268.

APPENDICES

A   Biological Meaning of the Restriction Term

To see how the restriction term in the Hamiltonian given by Eq. (1) is actually derived from the assumption of synaptic competition, I assume that the limited amount of factors synthesized at the presynaptic cell body per unit time might bring about the struggle for existence among the synaptic terminals of individual presynaptic neurons. This effect can be mathematically expressed as $-r\rho_{j,k,\mu_1\mu_2}\sum_{j'}\rho_{j',k,\mu_1,\mu_2}$ and added to the right-hand side of the dynamic equation for synaptic connections as follows:

$$(A1) \quad \frac{d}{dt}\rho_{j,k,\mu_1,\mu_2} = \rho_{j,k,\mu_1,\mu_2}\left[1 - \sum_{k',\mu_1',\mu_2'}\rho_{j,k',\mu_1',\mu_2'} - g\zeta_j\eta_{k,\mu_1,\mu_2}\right.$$
$$\left. -r\sum_{j'}\rho_{j',k,\mu_1,\mu_2}\right] + \varepsilon_{j,k,\mu_1,\mu_2}.$$

According to the thermodynamic reformulation of steady-state solutions to this equation, which has been fully discussed in a previous paper [40], we can obtain a modified energy function which includes the effect of competition among synaptic terminals of individual presynaptic neurons,

$$(A2) \quad H = -\sum_j\sum_{k,\mu_1,\mu_2}\sigma_{j,k,\mu_1,\mu_2}\left[\langle\zeta_j\eta_{k,\mu_1,\mu_2}\rangle - \frac{r}{g}\sum_{j'}\sigma_{j',k,\mu_1,\mu_2}\right]$$
$$+\varepsilon_{j,k,\mu_1,\mu_2},$$

where $<>$ represents the ensemble average with respect to the fluctuation $\delta\eta_{k,\mu_1,\mu_2}$. Using the fact that the total number of synaptic connections

$\sum_{k,\mu_1,\mu_2}\sum_j \sigma_{j,k,\mu_1\mu_2}$ takes a constant value $4\bar{n}M$, where M is the total number of presynaptic neurons, Eq. (1) is obtained. Therefore, the coefficient c of the restriction term in Eq. (1) corresponds to the ratio r/g. In this transformation, the constant terms in the Hamiltonian can be omitted, since they do not affect the formation of synaptic connections. In this way, the restriction term in the Hamiltonian turns out to be derived from the assumption of synaptic competition due to the limited amount of factors from individual presynaptic neurons.

B   Derivation of the presynaptic correlation function

When visual stimulation is presented to the retina, the signal is transferred in a nonlinear manner. However, if we apply the linearization procedure, the fluctuation in retinal ganglion cell activity $\delta\eta^G_{k,\mu_1,\mu_2}$ is proportional to the fluctuation in membrane potential of the photoreceptor cell $\delta\zeta^P_{m,\mu_1,\mu_2}$ as follows:

$$(\text{B1}) \qquad \delta\eta^G_{k,\mu_1,\mu_2} = \sum_m \mu_2 R^G_{k;m}\delta\zeta^P_{m,\mu_1,\mu_2}.$$

Function $R^G_{k;m}$ represents the RF of the ganglion cell at position k. Since retinal ganglion cells have concentric and center-surround antagonistic RFs, the ON-center presynaptic RF profile is modeled by Eq. (5).

The correlation function between any pair of ganglion cells is given by

$$(\text{B2}) \qquad \Gamma^{pre}_{k,\mu_1,\mu_2;k',\mu_1',\mu_2'} = \langle \delta\eta^G_{k,\mu_1,\mu_2}\delta\eta^G_{k',\mu_1',\mu_2'}\rangle.$$

In the absence of binocular form vision, one candidate for the origin of retinal ganglion cell firing is the unorganized spontaneous membrane polarization of photoreceptor cells. Therefore, the fluctuation in membrane potential $\delta\zeta^P_{m,\mu_1,\mu_2}$ is assumed to be Gaussian stochastic processes, in which the average and covariance are given by

$$(\text{B3}) \qquad \langle \delta\zeta^P_{m,\mu_1,\mu_2}\rangle = 0$$

$$(\text{B4}) \qquad \langle \delta\zeta^P_{m,\,\mu_1,\mu_2}\delta\zeta^P_{m',\mu_1',\mu_2'}\rangle = \delta_{m,m'}\delta_{\mu_1,\mu_1'}\delta_{\mu_2,\mu_2'}.$$

Here, the delta function $\delta_{m,m'}$ indicates the stochastic independence between neural activities of photoreceptors located separately. $\delta_{\mu_1,\mu_1'}$

indicates the absence of interactions between pathways originating in the left and right eyes. Combining Eqs. (B1), (B2) and (B4), the presynaptic correlation function $\Gamma^{pre}_{k,\mu_1,\mu_2;k',\mu'_1,\mu'_2}$ is rewritten as

$$(B5) \qquad \Gamma^{pre}_{k,\mu_1,\mu_2;k',\mu'_1,\mu'_2} = 2\gamma^P \delta_{\mu_1,\mu'_1} \mu_2 \mu'_2 C^{GG}_{k;k'},$$

where $C^{GG}_{k;k'}$ is calculated from the convolution of the presynaptic RF function $R^G_{k;m}$ as follows:

$$(B6) \qquad C^{GG}_{k;k'} = \sum_m R^G_{k;m} R^G_{k';m}.$$

C   Derivation of the Cortical Receptive Field

We simulated responses of model visual cortical neurons to the presentation of light or dark oriented bars at various positions in the visual field (Fig. 1), using synaptic connections which were self-organized based on our thermodynamic theory without binocular form vision. The firing rate of the model cortical neuron η_j is expressed by

$$(C1) \qquad \eta_j = F\left(\sum_{k,\mu_1,\mu_2} \sum_{j'} \sum_m V^{post}_{j;j'} \sigma_{j',k,\mu_1,\mu_2} \mu_2 R^G_{k;m} S_{m,\mu_1} - \zeta^{th} \right).$$

This formula is interpreted in the following way. First, the stimulus S_{m,μ_1} presented at the position m in the retina specified by ocularity μ_1 is received by the retinal ganglion cell through its concentric RF $\mu_2 R^G_{k;m}$ where $\mu_2 = +1$ for ON-center presynaptic neurons and $\mu_2 = -1$ for OFF-center neurons. Then the firing of the ganglion cell induced by the stimulus is transferred to cortical neurons through the self-organized afferent synaptic connections $\{\sigma_{j,k,\mu_1,\mu_2}\}$. As these presynaptic firings are gathered through the dendritic and intracortical connections represented by $V^{post}_{j;j'}$, the membrane potential of the cortical neuron is depolarized, and finally the neuron fires. Here, the stimulus function S_{m,μ_1} is chosen to be a step function which takes a non-zero value only within a rectangular area and is zero outside. The non-zero value is positive for the light bar stimulus, whereas it is negative for the dark bar. Nonlinearity in the transformation from membrane potential to firing rate is described by the function F such that $F(x) = x$ for $x \geq 0$; $F(x) = 0$ otherwise. The parameter ζ^{th} represents the membrane potential at the threshold of firing. Then we linearize Eq. (C1), by considering the fluctuation in activity of the cortical neuron $\delta\eta_j$ in response to the fluctuation in stimulus intensity $\delta S_{m,\mu_1}$. The monocular RF function R^{VC}_{j,m,μ_1} is defined by

$$(\text{C2}) \qquad \delta\eta_j = \sum_{\mu_1}\sum_m R^{VC}_{j,m,\mu_1}\,\delta S_{m,\mu_1}.$$

Here, $\delta S_{m,\mu_1}$ represents the intensity fluctuation of the light stimulus presented to the position m in the retina specified by ocularity μ_1. $\delta\eta_j$ represents the fluctuation in the activity of the cortical neuron at position j in response to the stimulus. Comparing Eq. (C1) with Eq. (C2), we can obtain the following formula for the visual cortical RF:

$$(\text{C3}) \qquad R^{VC}_{j,m,\mu_1} \propto \sum_{j'}\sum_{\mu_2'}\sum_{k'} V^{post}_{j;j'}\,\sigma_{j',k',\mu_1,\mu_2'}\,\mu_2'\,R^{G}_{k';m}.$$

Since we are not interested in the absolute magnitude of the cortical RFs, the proportionality is replaced by the equality in Eq. (C3).

Chapter 6
A Neuroidal Model for Cognition

Leslie G. Valiant*

1   Introduction

Over the last century experimental psychologists have discovered a wide
range of cognitive phenomena in humans and other species. Many of these
phenomena have proved impressively robust and reproducible. Experimental
findings relating to these phenomena are accumulating at a rapid pace, and
the problem of finding theories that explain broad ranges of them has become
more and more urgent. Theories are needed to summarize and communicate
existing findings and also to predict new ones.

Successful theories of particular groups of findings exist but the question
nevertheless arises as to why none of these has proved more successful in
explaining broader ranges of phenomena. The answer we shall suggest is
that most of these theories are perhaps just too simple. Theories that are a
little more detailed may be needed. As an analogy one might consider the
case of high school mathematics, which can be applied to provide piecemeal
theories of a wide range of real world phenomena. In order to capture the
most general theories of physics, however, models are needed that are one
or two levels more complex.

In this paper we shall advocate a style of computational modeling
based on *neuroids*. This model was developed to bridge the gap between
computations at the neural level, and the functionality of biological systems
at the cognitive level. A neuroid is similar to a classical threshold element
as defined by McCulloch and Pitts [6] except that it is augmented with
states. The availability of these extra states makes the model more flexibly
programmable than conventional neural network models. The model is
intended to be used as a language in which a wide range of theories of the
mechanisms that underlie cognition can be described and studied. It enables
such mechanisms to be specified in terms of three things: the programs
that execute on each neuroid, the nature of the *network* that interconnects
the neuroids, and the interfaces the system has with any *peripheral* devices
that perform input/output or other auxiliary functions. The model is not
committed to any single algorithmic process.

A major goal of this model is to provide a basis on which the algorithmic

*Aiken Computation Laboratory, Harvard University, Cambridge, MA 02138

feasibility of well defined idealizations of cognitive functions can be studied. In particular the model allows one to quantify the resources needed by computations in terms of the number of steps, the number of neuroids, and the degree of connectivity of the network. The model has been used to explore algorithms for a class of tasks, called *random access tasks* that appear to test the constraints the most severely. These tasks can be characterized as those that, in each new invocation, may potentially require access to any part of the information already stored in memory. Examples are the memorization of an item that is related to previously memorized items, the recall of an item from memory, forming a new association and inductive learning of concepts.

This model may be studied from any one of several perspectives. One may, for example, attempt to glean new insights into the nature of cognition by investigating the limits of what is computationally feasible on brain-like models of computation. Alternatively, one can use any such insights gained as a starting point, and investigate new mechanisms for simulating significant aspects of cognition by machine. This paper, which is expository in nature and aimed at a computer science audience, is devoted entirely to a third motivation which can be summarized by the following question: Is the neuroidal model a useful model for formulating theories in cognitive science?

2   An Outline of the Neuroidal Model

We shall outline the model in terms of its three major aspects. A fuller account of these can be found elsewhere [12].

(1) A neuroidal system consists of a network of *neuroids*. Each neuroid can be viewed as a threshold element that at any time is in one of a finite number of allowed *states*. Some states are considered to be firing states, while others are not. The neuroid has two transition functions defined. The first, called δ, specifies the updates to the state and threshold in terms of three parameters: the previous state, the previous threshold, and the sum of the weights of all edges incoming from neuroids that are in a firing state. The second transition function, called λ, specifies how each weight is updated as a function of five parameters: its previous weight, the firing status of the neighbor it is coming from, and, in addition, the three parameters that influence the first transition δ. By means of these two kinds of transitions one can program neuroids in a flexible way. In particular, one can incorporate a variety of timing mechanisms that lend power to the model.

(2) The neuroidal model of computation may support diverse styles of computation. There is, however, essentially one style for which substantial functionality has been already demonstrated. This is based on what we call *positive* knowledge representations. A positive representation is discrete, hierarchical and, because of connectivity limitations, graded. At the most basic level a semantic unit or *item* is represented by about r neuroids where r

is called the replication factor. An item may represent, among other things, a concept such as "yellow", an individual object, person or event, or some lower level perceptual unit. When the item is *recognized* by the system all or most of the neuroids that represent it fire. In general, except for items that are preprogrammed, just those items are added to the memory that are experienced and attended to. By ensuring that in each experience only a bounded number of neuroids are allocated, one can guarantee that the total number of neuroids ever needed is no more than proportional to the lifetime of the system.

The combined nature of the network and of the programs in the neuroids is such that they jointly support several *basic functions.* If A and B are items already represented then an execution of the function JOIN will allocate about r previously unused neuroids to the conjunction "A and B" in the sense that at later times these neuroids will fire whenever the neuroids representing A and those representing B all fire. An execution of a second function LINK on a pair of items A,B will have the different effect that whenever A fires in the future, so will B. The network may be such that either of these two effects is obtained equally for every pair A,B. Alternatively it may be divided into areas, much as the cortex is believed to be, so that these effects are obtained preferentially for pairs of items stored within areas having some degree of proximity to each other.

The neuroids have implemented on them a variety of programs that realize idealizations of cognitive functions. Using as building blocks JOIN, which implements memory allocation, and LINK, which implements a form of association, a variety of memorization, inductive learning and correlation detection algorithms can be supported. Furthermore, this range of functionalities is supported together compatibly within a single system, so that each invocation of any one does not disturb the results of previous invocations.

(3) The issues discussed so far can be defined and discussed within a simple precise formal model. We may wish to go outside this model, however, for at least two purposes. First, we may wish to discuss how the neuroidal system interacts with its peripheral systems by describing its interfaces but without specifying how the interfaces themselves are realized by these other systems. Second, the neuroid transitions as defined are designed to support the implementation of the most important random access tasks in the simplest way. We may wish to complicate the model in various ways to model aspects of biology more closely.

We shall show in the next section how this model can be used to describe theories to explain various aspects of the basic phenomena of Pavlovian conditioning. We shall not discuss the model itself in any more technical detail here. We note merely that reference [12] provides further discussion of many of the issues we have briefly hinted at here.

The one feature of the model that we wish, however, to highlight here is that positive results are available regarding its theoretical underpinnings. These underpinnings are of various forms: specifications of the neuroidal programs that implement the claimed tasks, specifications of the connectivity properties that are required of the network by these various programs, demonstrations that the computations on this model can be simulated efficiently on models that resemble biological neurons and connectivity more closely, and demonstrations that some idealizations of higher level tasks such as reasoning, and processing relational information, can be supported on the model also. These underpinnings provide a basis for investigating network theories of neural functions. They confirm the computational feasibility of maintaining data structures of exactly this kind, by mechanisms that can be executed on a brain-like model of computation. Furthermore, they provide specific meanings to the diagrams, such as Figure 1 below, that go beyond those of conventional graph based methods of representing knowledge.

3   Pavlovian Conditioning

Pavlovian conditioning is a phenomenon in which the behavior of an organism is modified in a particular manner by means of a particular procedure. It is based invariably on the existence of a stimulus that unconditionally provokes a certain response. Thus a puff of air in the eye of an animal will cause it to blink. The air puff is called the *unconditioned stimulus* US, and the blinking is the *unconditioned response* UR. Based on this pair (US,UR) the process of Pavlovian conditioning can be used to make the organism produce a response CR similar to UR (i.e. blinking in this case) when an unrelated stimulus, such as the sight of a yellow square, is presented. The method of achieving this conditioning is to subject the organism to a long series of trials in each of which the chosen *conditioned stimulus* CR, the yellow square in this case, and the US, or air puff, are presented together in a certain manner. Each such training trial will evoke the UR since the US is present. The final outcome of a long enough sequence of such training trials is that if the CS, the yellow square, is presented now *even in the absence* of the US, the air puff, the CR, or blinking, will result nevertheless.

The phenomenon of Pavlovian conditioning is an ideal target for neuroidal modelling for several reasons. First, there already exists an exceptionally large body of coherent experimental data relating to this phenomenon. Second, we argue that if it should happen that there *is* an instance of the neuroidal model that is a good general model of cognition, then Pavlovian conditioning offers an ideal experimental tool for uncovering the details of this instance. Such experiments should enable one to tease apart the internal workings of the proverbial "black box" that exhibits the cognitive behaviors. Thirdly, the neuroidal model is compatible with some of the notions in terms of which Pavlovian conditioning is discussed in the existing psychology literature. In particular the notion that a set of neuroids represents a semantic item can be interpreted as similar to Pavlov's less formal notion of a "center" [7]. Furthermore the inductive learning algorithms that can be programmed on neuroids include those, such as the Rescorla-Wagner model, that have been proposed and tested extensively in the Pavlovian context [9]. We take some encouragement from this fact that existing psychological thinking in at least one area of cognition is already sympathetic to the neuroidal model. Alternative proposals for unified theories of cognition, we would argue, do not fit any specific cognitive phenomenon quite so well. Methodological questions do remain, nevertheless, even in this limited domain. It is not clear, for example, that the phenomena that fit the Rescorla-Wagner model reflect the properties of single neurons, rather than more complex assemblies of them. Also, while it appears that the cerebral cortex has a role in conditioning when the conditioned stimulus is complex, a variety of other parts of the brain are also involved that depend on the nature of the stimulus. These other parts may use different kinds of neurons.

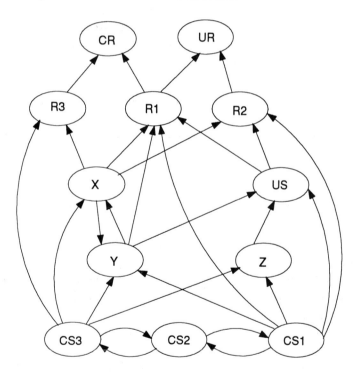

Schematic diagram showing a number of items and some associations between certain pairs of them. Each ellipse represents an item. Each directed edge represents an influence that exceeds some minimum strength.

We shall now enumerate some of the basic phenomena of Pavlovian conditioning and show how they can be expressed in terms of the neuroidal model. Further details about them can be found in the literature (e.g. [5, 7]). First we consider a schematic fragment of a neuroidal circuit that is shown in Figure 1. Each item is represented schematically by an ellipse. A directed line from one ellipse to another represents a possibly large number of connections from the nodes of the first item to the nodes of the second. Such a line is shown only for those of the physical connections that have high enough weight that the firing of the first item will cause the second to fire, or, at least, bring it significantly closer to firing. Note that some connections may be realized via intermediate relay neuroids that are not shown. Figure 1, in other words, can be viewed as summarizing the strong associations that exist among the items shown.

In the figure the items are given various suggestive names.   US corresponds to the unconditioned stimulus, and we assume that in the initial condition of the network its firing will cause the items R1 and R2 to fire, which together we shall regard as initiating the unconditioned response UR. CS1, CS2 and CS3 are items that are used as conditioned stimuli in various combinations in the different experiments. In the course of trials that control these items from the outside, various connections may be established among them as well as between them and some further items, such as X,Y or Z, which are somehow close by in the network. The particular network of associations that arises is a function of several parameters: the programs in the individual neuroids, the topology of the underlying network, the initial conditions, and the sequence of training trials to which the system has been subject.

We shall consider the various phenomena in three groups, according to which of the aspects of the neuroidal model they emphasize most: (i) connectivity and knowledge representation, (ii) inductive learning, or (iii) timing phenomena. The idea we are trying to suggest is that by taking into consideration the large body of existing experimental findings, and by performing new experiments as necessary, one can hope to discover detailed and reliable models that capture in a unified way much of the diversity of the known phenomena.

In the first group we shall consider five phenomena. *Classical conditioning* is the simplest form of Pavlovian conditioning and is the one we have already described. In terms of Figure 1 we can regard CS1 as being the conditioned stimulus (the yellow square), US as the unconditioned stimulus (the air puff) and UR the response (blinking). Classical conditioning, at the first level, can be accounted for as the establishment of a LINK operation either from CS1 to CR or from CS1 to US, or perhaps a combination of both. The question of which of these viewpoints offers the best explanation has been investigated at length. Experiments suggest that for each viewpoint circumstances can be found in which it is the most plausible.

Second order conditioning is a phenomenon that is achieved as a result of two phases of classical conditioning. First CS1 is paired with US to achieve conditioning as above. In a subsequent phase a second stimulus CS2 is paired with CS1, each time also evoking CR by virtue of the initial conditioning. The final result achieved after these two phases is that CS2 alone will evoke a response CR. This can be explained in various ways. A LINK connection may be established CS2 $\rightarrow$ CS1. Alternatively it may be established CS2 $\rightarrow$ US or even CS $\rightarrow$ CR. Evidence for each of these mechanisms can be found, depending on the conditions. For example, if CS1 and CS2 are semantically closely related then it appears that the CS2 $\rightarrow$ CS1 connection is favored [8]. We also note that conditioning can be chained even beyond second order. For example, third order conditioning has been reported.

Sensory preconditioning achieves the same result as second order conditioning, and consists of the same two phases but in reverse order. Thus in the first phase CS2 and CS1 are paired, and no response evoked, while in the second phase CS1 and US are paired.

Some *variation* between the CR and the UR is usually found in classical conditioning. While the response evoked by the conditioned stimulus is similar to that evoked by the unconditioned stimulus, it is not identical. For example, the blinking may differ in intensity or in other qualitative aspects. This variation phenomenon may be explained by the fact suggested in Figure 1, that since LINK connections can be realized between arbitrary pairs of items that fire at appropriate times, as the circuit becomes more complex more and more indirect connections and unexpected side-effects may result. Hence, although conditioning may establish a new LINK from CS1 to US or from CS1 to nodes on the pathway to UR, there is no guarantee that the result will be that the firing of CS1 and of US will cause the various nodes of UR to fire at exactly the same strengths. Hence this variation is exactly what one would expect from a neuroidal model once the strong connections in the network become complex.

Generalization is the phenomenon in which, after classical conditioning with CS1, a stimulus CS3 similar to CS1 but not identical to it, will also produce a response similar to CR. A neuroidal explanation of this is that because of the similarity between CS1 and CS3 there are some nodes that are excited by both. In Figure 1 examples of these are shown as Y and Z. Then conditioning by CS3 can be expected to set up LINKs to US or CR from these same nodes, Y or Z, exactly as does conditioning by CS1.

We claim that these phenomena taken together are suggestive of an underlying system that resembles the way in which a neuroidal system supports random access functions. In particular, classical conditioning appears to be able to set up connections between arbitrary pairs of items. Furthermore, the outcome of a succession of conditioning experiments appears to be consistent with the expected effects of the chains of connections that would be set up in the model.

We shall now consider the second group of phenomena, which can be regarded as relating particularly to the basic *inductive learning* algorithms used by neurons. The question here is: What rules govern the weight changes that neurons undergo as a function of training? In the neuroidal model different neuroids may execute different algorithms by virtue of being in different states. Some neuroids may be initialized to be able to memorize one event or individual, and may be immutable once they have performed this act. Others may be initialized to induce a concept or function from a long sequence of examples. Here we shall consider this latter case. For simplicity we shall assume that the experimental results described are all manifestations of the same neural algorithm.

For describing these experiments we shall use the following notation that is adapted from one used in the literature. We assume that the same US, UR pair is used throughout, and in each trial we shall indicate + or − according to whether in that trial the US is or is not used. Thus A+ will denote classical conditioning with conditioned stimulus A, and AB+ will denote the same but in which two stimuli A,B are presented simultaneously instead of just one. We optionally put parentheses around the description of a phase of training where this provides clarity. Thus {A+}{B+} indicates two phases of classical conditioning, first with conditioned stimulus A, and subsequently with stimulus B. {A+, B+} will denote a single phase where the two stimuli are randomly mixed, to distinguish it from {AB+} in which both stimuli are presented at every trial. The influence of a conditioned stimulus A on CR we shall denote by a number W_A, (to suggest the weight of an edge from A to the response item in the idealization that there is just one such connection that is furthermore direct).

Using this notation we describe classical conditioning as

$$A+ \; \Rightarrow \; W_A \uparrow .$$

In general, the lefthand side describes the training phase or phases, and the righthand side the final outcome, in this case the change in value of W_A. We will denote such changes by $\uparrow, \downarrow$ and $=$ indicating whether the quantity increases, decreases, or remains unchanged, respectively, as a result of the phases described.

Some of the basic phenomena that shed light on inductive learning can be summarized qualitatively as follows. *Extinction* is the phenomenon in which after a phase of classical conditioning with A, if in a second phase A is presented in the absence of the US, then A will eventually cease to evoke CR. In describing the A+ initialization condition, we will place it at the beginning of the expression in *square* brackets to denote that it is a precondition, rather than a constituent of the effect described. Thus

$$[A+]\{A-\} \; \Rightarrow \; W_A \downarrow .$$

means that if W_A has a certain value after a phase of classical conditioning, then this value will decrease if a phase of extinction then follows.

Subsequent to a classical conditioning phase, time alone has little effect:

$$[A+]\{-\} \;\Rightarrow\; W_A = .$$

Also reinforcement of the US subsequent to classical conditioning has little effect.

$$[A+]\{+\} \;\Rightarrow\; W_A = .$$

There are certain simple schedules in which the result of classical conditioning can be influenced by a prior phase. *CS pre-exposure* is the phenomenon in which $[A-]\{A+\}$ produces a smaller W_A than $\{A+\}$ alone. In *US pre-exposure*, $[+]\{A+\}$ produces a smaller W_A than $\{A+\}$ alone.

More complex phenomena can be exhibited if two conditioned stimuli, say A and B, are used rather than one. These may be in different modalities. Thus A may be a visual image and B an auditory tone. *Conditioned inhibition*,

$$\{A+, AB-\} \;\Rightarrow\; W_A \uparrow, W_B < 0,$$

arises from a training phase in which A+ and AB− trials are intermingled. The result of this training is that A alone will evoke CR, but B will not. Experiments suggest that the final effect of B is truly inhibitory in the sense that B acquires an ability to inhibit an unrelated stimulus C in the following sense: If such a stimulus C has been conditioned to evoke CR, it is found that presenting B and C together will produce a smaller response than C alone.

The *blocking effect* is

$$\{A+\}\{AB+\} \;\Rightarrow\; W_A \uparrow, W_B = .$$

The customary interpretation is that once A has been conditioned to evoke CR, the response CR is expected when A and B are presented together, and no further learning takes place.

The *overexpectation effect* is

$$[A+, B+]\{AB+\} \;\Rightarrow\; W_A \downarrow, W_B \downarrow.$$

Once either A or B can evoke CR, their presentation together will evoke a quantitative expectation of CR that is higher than the true value of CR, and some diminution of each of their individual influences will result.

A model that has proved to fit many but not all of these phenomena is the Rescorla-Wagner model [9]. In our terminology it can be formulated in a simplified way as follows. The US is given a *value* of 1 when it is present and 0 when it is not. Each CS, say A_i, has a strength of influence of W_{A_i} on the fixed response. The aim of the learning process is, roughly that for each combination of the A_i presented, the sum W of the W_{A_i} for just those A_i that are present, should predict correctly the value of the US (i.e. whether $US=0$ or $US=1$). The mechanism that achieves this that is hypothesized is the following:

1. Each W_{A_i} is unchanged in any trial in which $W=US$, (i.e. the existing weights predict correctly). It is also unchanged in any trial in which that particular A_i is not present.

2. If A_i is present in the trial then A_i is increased if $W < US$ and decreased if $W > US$. These increases or decreases are proportional to the magnitude of the difference between W and US.

There are several related models, such as the perceptron algorithm and the least mean squares rule, that are also based on the idea that in each trial the W_{A_i} need to be updated so that some linear combination of their values correctly predicts the response in some sense. Each of them can be adapted to explain many of the phenomena though not all, and we shall not enter into a full discussion of them here [1, 2, 3, 10, 11]. Perhaps the main distinguishing features of the neuroidal approach are that (1) it provides an integrated view of both the network properties *and* the neuroidal updates and (2) it proposes to model cognitive phenomena in some generality, rather than just for one class of experimental results. We shall, therefore, draw attention to two of the phenomena for which such a broader approach provides some natural explanations.

First, consider the CS pre-exposure effect. This is not explained by the standard version of the Rescorla-Wagner model that assumes that before any training each $W_{A_i} = 0$, and consequently predicts that $\{A_i-\}$ has no effect since $W = US = 0$ throughout such a preliminary phase. In the neuroidal approach it is natural to consider that the A_i neuroids and the US or UR neuroids are not connected physically directly, since the network is sparse. The connections that need to be strengthened are indirect, and go through intermediate neuroids. For these indirect connections to be established, some of the connections leaving the A_i neuroids need to be positive rather than zero at the start. In that case a natural explanation of the CS pre-exposure effect is that pre-exposure causes these weights to decrease, thus making it more difficult for any subsequent $\{A_i+\}$ phase to achieve conditioning. An alternative natural explanation, also implicit in the neuroidal model is that each synapse has fixed-sign, in the sense that the corresponding weight cannot change sign. Thus a typical weight may be always positive, with a multiplicative, rather than additive, update rule as in Littlestone's winnow algorithm [13]. In that case preexposure may have the effect of reducing the weight to so close to zero that it takes very many interactions to restore it later to a significant value.

A second finding that is not consistent with the Rescorla-Wagner model, or any other model that treats positive and negative values of

W_A symmetrically, is that, schedules that extinguish positive W_A do not necessarily do the same for negative W_A. In particular, an excitatory W_A can be extinguished by a $\{A-\}$ session, but an inhibitory W_A is typically left unchanged by $\{A-\}$. A natural way to approach this dilemma is to consider variations of the neuroidal update rule that are asymmetric in a biologically plausible way. In particular, it may be reasonable to consider a lower bound on W, the sum of the A_i, so that values below this bound are indistinguishable. For example, if this bound is zero, then part (2) of the Rescorla-Wagner rule can be modified so that A_i is increased only if $W < US$ and $W \geq 0$. Such a modification has been proposed before to the Rescorla-Wagner model in order to fit this same phenomenon (e.g.[11]). Our point here is that this modification fits a very natural definition of neuroids, and if so interpreted has potentially verifiable consequences for cognition beyond Pavlovian conditioning.

We also note that explanations in the literature of Pavlovian phenomena even in this second group, often appeal to network phenomena implicitly. For example, when there are two conditioned stimuli being considered, the issue often arises of whether, besides the separate centers for A and B, a center for "A and B" also exists.

Finally, we discuss a third category of phenomena that are related to *time* in various ways. The first of these relates to the *conditioning schedule*. We asserted above that to obtain classical conditioning the CS and the US need to be presented together in some way. In fact, the strength of the effect obtained appears to depend critically on the relative timing of these two stimuli. In particular, the response is largest if the onset of the CS is slightly prior to the onset of the US. If the stimuli are simultaneous, or separated by too large an interval, then the conditioning effect is small or nonexistent. One might say that, if a CS is followed by a US, then it is reasonable for an organism to interpret the US as being the consequence of the CS, and hence to *expect* the US on being exposed to the CS. We note that in many of the applications that we have worked out for the neuroidal model timing is used carefully in the encoding of inputs. Hence the criticality of timing in the corresponding psychological phenomena is only to be expected.

A second effect is *spontaneous recovery*. If in a succession of days an animal is exposed to a sequence of extinction trials, it is found that each morning the conditioned response has partially recovered as compared to the level of extinction reached at the end of the previous day. This can be interpreted as implying that recent changes to weights have a tendency to partially decay with time towards the level that held prior to these changes. The neuroidal model can be extended easily to capture this kind of time dependence.

Yet another category of time dependent effects, that include *external inhibition* and *external disinhibition*, occur when during the acquisition phase or during an extinction phase, respectively, some novel stimulus is presented just prior to the presentation of the CS. The effect in either case is as if the subject were distracted by the novel stimulus, and regresses to the behavior that would have been expected prior to the current training phase. Thus during classical conditioning the novel stimulus will prevent the CS from evoking CR, while during extinction it will have the result that the CS will evoke the CR as if no extinction had taken place. In the former case of external inhibition, the explanation that the novel stimulus simply diverts attention from the CS is plausible. In the latter case of external disinhibition a more subtle explanation is needed. Pavlov's theory was essentially that extinction involved not merely the reduction in a positive weight, but the increase in strength of a separate connection that was inhibitory and, further, that such inhibitory connections were brittle when first established and therefore easily disrupted. In the neuroidal model it is natural to entertain such "temporarily brittle connections." Unless the network properties are ideal, the task of establishing a new connection by means of LINK is not trivial. Some theories of the brain suggest that long term memory is laid down in the course of several weeks or months, as a result of repeated rehearsals, effected by such mechanisms as the hippocampus. These rehearsals are necessary to make long term associations as robust and effective as the memories that are already permanent.

4   Conclusion

In the previous section we have attempted to suggest that the neuroidal model may be a useful model for formulating detailed theories of Pavlovian conditioning. There are a number of other psychological phenomena for which one could make a similar argument. Priming [4] is discussed in [12]. It is suggested there that a plausible starting point for a detailed neuroidal theory of these phenomena is the simple theory that priming effects are due to temporary increases in weights.

The advantage of having cognitive theories as detailed as those that can be expressed in the neuroidal model is that one should be able to resolve among them by experimentation more conclusively than among theories that have inherently insufficient detail. More detailed theories will, of course, need more supportive evidence to be convincingly corroborated. But this is an unavoidable cost whenever the underlying phenomena have sufficient inherent complexity.

There is also the broader issue of whether corroboration of the value of the neuroidal model for understanding cognition in some generality can be obtained by examining only a small number of very specific phenomena. We suspect that if this is indeed possible then Pavolvian conditioning may be a fruitful vehicle for such a pursuit.

References

[1] R. ATKINSON, et. al. (eds), *Stevens' Handbook of Experimental Psychology*, Wiley, New York, 2nd ed., 1988.

[2] N. DONEGAN, M. GLUCK, AND R. THOMPSON, *Integrating behavioral and biological models of classical conditioning*, The Psychology of Learning and Motivation, 23 (1989), pp. 109–156.

[3] M. GLUCK AND G. BOWER, *Evaluating an adaptive network model of human learning*, Journal of Memory and Language, 27 (1988), pp. 166–195.

[4] P. GRAF AND M. MASSON, *Implicit Memory*. Lawrence Erlbaum, P. Graf and M.E. Masson, eds., Hillsdale, NJ, 1993.

[5] J. MAZUR, *Learning and Behavior*, 1990. Prentice Hall , Englewood, Cliffs, NJ.

[6] W. MCCULLOCH AND W. PITTS, *A logical calculus of ideas immanent in nervous activity*, Bull. of Math. Biophysics, (5)115 (1943).

[7] I. PAVLOV, *Lectures on Conditioned Reflexes*. International Publishers, New York, 1928.

[8] R. RESCORLA, *Three Pavlovian paradigms*, in Primary Neural Substrates of Learning and Behavioral Change, D. Alkon and J. Farley, eds., Cambridge University Press, 1982.

[9] R. RESCORLA AND A. WAGNER, *A theory of Pavlovian conditioning: Variations in the effectiveness of reinforcement and nonreinforcement.* In Classical Conditioning II: Current research and theory, Appleton-Century-Crofts, A. Black and W.F. Prokasy, eds., New York, 1972.

[10] R. SUTTON AND A. BARTO, *Toward a modern theory of adaptive networks: Expectation and prediction*, Psych. Rev., 88 (1981), pp. 135–170.

[11] R. SUTTON AND A. BARTO, *A temporal-difference model of classical conditioning.*, in Proc. 9th Ann. Conf. of the Cognitive Science Society, Seattle, WA, 1987, pp. 355–378.

[12] L. VALIANT, *Circuits of the Mind*. Oxford University Press, New York, 1994.

[13] N. LITTLESTONE, *Learning Quickly When Irrelevant Attributes Abound: A New Linear Threshold Algorithm.*, in Machine Learning, 2(4):285-318, 1988.

Chapter 7
Knowledge Discovery in Genetic Sequences

Akihiko Konagaya*

Abstract

The effectiveness of a stochastic approach for analyzing genetic information such as DNA sequences and protein sequences is described. AI technologies, especially machine learning technologies, can be extremely effective for extracting valuable information from the enormous amounts of genetic sequences generated by biologists. To achieve this, however, more flexible and robust learning methodologies are required to deal with diversity occurring in the genetic sequences. In this paper, we show how a stochastic approach, including stochastic knowledge representations and stochastic learning algorithms, works for knowledge discovery in genetic sequences using a system we call motif extraction as an example. The motif extraction system aims to extract stable common patterns (motifs) conserved in the evolutional process. In the system, motifs are regarded as stochastic rules, and a genetic algorithm with Rissanen's minimum description length (MDL) principle is used as a learning algorithm. The MDL principle enables us to select "good stochastic motifs" from the viewpoint of balancing the complexity of the motif and its fitness to training data. This paper also briefly describes some instances of extracting stochastic motifs from super families in a protein data base (PIR), the comparison of the MDL principle and the maximum likelihood method in terms of genetic algorithms, and the Hidden Markov Model (HMM) representation of stochastic motifs.

1 Introduction

Recent molecular biology enables us to discover genetic information in chromosomes such as DNA sequences and protein sequences. Since the amount of genetic sequence data is so large, it is impossible to understand them without the help of computers. This has led to the birth of a new science called genetic information processing or bioinformatics.

Although genetic information processing covers a wide area including genetic sequence database systems, homology search systems and protein structure estimation, one of the most important and exciting areas is knowledge discovery in genetic sequences such as motif extraction. In this

---

*Computer System Research Laboratory, C&C Research Laboratories, NEC Corporation.

paper, *motif*, in biological terms, means an evolutionarily preserved pattern in protein sequences with the same function or structure[1, 2]. This paper mainly focuses on the extraction of motifs from protein sequences and shows the effectiveness of stochastic AI technologies to deal with noise in genetic sequences caused by divergence.

Divergence is one of the most important characteristics of creatures. In fact, it seems difficult to find a rule without exceptions for creatures. One such instance is a rule to distinguish birds from mammals. One may say that birds have bills, lay eggs and have feathers or wings, and mammals have four legs and bear babies. However, a duckbill has four legs and a bill, and lays eggs! Thus, rules in creatures should be a kind of approximation with some probability assigned, that is, stochastic rules.

The same problem occurs in knowledge discovery in genetic sequences especially for motif extraction. The purpose of motif extraction is to find a rule that distinguishes the target protein sequences from other sequences. From this point of view, it is natural to use machine learning techniques for motif extraction. However, it should be taken in account that the motif extraction requires a flexible and robust learning method to extract valuable information from a large number of sequences with noise.

The stochastic approach is one such method proposed by the author for motif extraction[6]. The characteristics of the stochastic approach are the use of stochastic representation of rules, stochastic search algorithms and quantitative criteria of stochastic rules. For instance, a motif (stochastic motif in this paper) is considered as a stochastic rule which represents a probabilistic relationship between a set of protein categories and genetic sequences. One such representation is a stochastic decision predicate which consists of Horn clauses with probabilities[5]. The Hidden Markov Model (HMM) is another example of a stochastic motif representation[4]. In order to avoid overfitting to the training sequences the MDL principle has been adopted as a quantitative criterion of stochastic motifs. The MDL principle enables us to select a stochastic motif that balances the complexity of the representation and its fitness to the training sequences. However, it is computationally intractable to find the exact MDL solution from the whole set of possible motifs. To solve the problem, a genetic algorithm has been adopted. The essense of our genetic algorithm is the use of the MDL principle in the design of a fitness function[7]. This methodology not only avoids overfitting to training sequences but also has proved that the MDL principle is effective for improving the convergent performance of genetic algorithms when it produces an appropriate bias on the fitness landscape. In addition, an asynchronous parallel genetic algorithm has been adopted to make effective use of parallel machines. In this algorithm, the population is divided into a set of subpopulations in which individuals migrate asynchronously. The migration overhead is negligible and 7.7 times speedup is observed when using 8 processors on a shared memory machine.

Species	Sequence of Cytochrome c
Human	..FIMKCSQCHTVEK..
Mouse	..FVQKCAQCHTVEK..
Chicken	..FVQKCSQCHTVEK..
Snake	..FSMKCGTCHTVEE..
Prawn	..FVQRCAQCHSAQA..
Yeast	..FKTRCLQCHTVEK..
Hemp	..FKTKCAECHTVGR..
Tetrahymena	..FDSQCSACHAIEG..
Rhodopila	..FHTICILCHTDIK..
Microbium	..VFKQCKICHQVGP..
Pseudomonas	..VFKQCMTCHRADK..

FIG. 1. *Some portions of cytochrome c sequences*

The organization of the rest of this paper is the following. Section 2 gives an introduction of motif extraction and describes why a stochastic extension of motifs is necessary. A representation for stochastic motifs, which we call *Stochastic Decision Predicates* is also described. Section 3 gives a strategy for selecting a good stochastic motif using the MDL principle. Section 4 gives a genetic algorithm for finding optimal stochastic motifs. Section 5 presents the experimental results on extracting stochastic motifs based on our methodology. Finally, in section 6 we discuss experimental results for our motif extraction system, the effectiveness of the MDL principle for GA convergence, and motif extraction using the HMM.

2   Stochastic Motifs

Motifs, in biological terms, mean common patterns in protein sequences that have been preserved in the evolutional process. In general, mutation probabilities on amino acids in a protein sequence are not uniform. It is often said that the more important the amino acids, the more conservative their evolution. This means that finding some conservative patterns in protein sequences provides some clues about the functions or structures of those proteins. In other words, the role of motif extraction is very similar to finding words in natural language.

Recently, some biologists and computer scientists have proposed various ways for extracting motifs [9, 10, 11]. However, no standard way is established so far even among biologists. The "stochastic motifs" described in this paper are one of the proposals for motif extraction.

A good example is a heme c binding site motif in a cytochrome c protein. Cytochrome c is one of the proteins that binds to a heme c which uses iron to transport electrons in creatures. It plays an important role in the respiratory chain and is famous as the first protein whose evolutionary tree

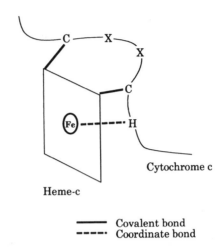

Heme-c

Cytochrome c

———— Covalent bond
----- Coordinate bond

FIG. 2. *A heme c binding in a cytochrome c*

was established by comparing protein sequences in various species. Figure 1 shows some portions of known cytochrome c sequences. Each character in the sequence corresponds to an amino acid. In most cytochrome c sequences, we can find the common pattern "CXXCH" which represents a cysteine, followed by two arbitrary amino acids, followed by another cysteine, followed by a histidine. In this pattern the second "X" does not necessarily coincide with the first "X". The pattern "CXXCH" can be considered as a motif for a cytochrome c, because it corresponds to a protein function; two cysteines and one histidine bind to a heme c which cytochrome c holds in the center (Figure 2).

As with other motifs, the pattern "CXXCH" also has exceptions. It does not exist in the cytochrome c of Euglena, and the pattern "CXXCH" exists in an adrenodoxin of a pig which is a different category from the cytochrome c. That is, the pattern "CXXCH" is just an indication of a heme c binding site of cytochrome c.

It is at this point that stochastic motifs differ from other approaches. Stochastic motifs represent the relationship between *protein function and/or structure*, and a *protein category* as posterior probabilities obtained from discriminate conditions. The following example gives the flavor of a stochastic motif. "If the pattern ⋯ "CXXCH" ⋯ is included in the sequence, then the sequence is cytochrome c with probability 137/244 and otherwise it belongs to other protein categories with probability 9386/9389." One representation of a stochastic motif is a stochastic decision predicate that consists of Horn clauses and their probability parameters as follows.

```
motif(S,cytochrome_c) with 137/244.
      :- contain(S,''CXXCH'').
motif(S,others) with 9386/9389.
```

The general form is the following.

$$motif(S, C_1) \quad \text{with } p_1 \quad :- Q_1^{(1)} \wedge \cdots \wedge Q_{k_1}^{(1)}.$$
$$motif(S, C_2) \quad \text{with } p_2 \quad :- Q_1^{(2)} \wedge \cdots \wedge Q_{k_2}^{(2)}.$$
$$\cdots\cdots\cdots\cdots$$
$$\cdots\cdots\cdots\cdots$$
$$motif(S, C_{m-1}) \text{ with } p_{m-1} :- Q_1^{(m-1)} \wedge \cdots \wedge Q_{k_{m-1}}^{(m-1)}.$$
$$motif(S, C_m) \quad \text{with } p_m \quad :- Q_1^{(m)} \wedge \cdots \wedge Q_{k_m}^{(m)}.$$

Here we call each "$motif(S, C_i)$ with p_i $:- Q_1^{(i)} \wedge \cdots \wedge Q_{k_i}^{(i)}$." a *stochastic clause*. The stochastic clause can be read: "Sequence S is in category C_i with probability p_i if $Q_1^{(i)}, \cdots, Q_{k_i}^{(i)}$ are all **true**". We assume sequential interpretation of the stochastic clauses in this paper. That is, $motif(S, C_i)$ is tested only after $motif(S, C_1), \cdots, motif(S, C_{i-1})$ have been tested and failed. The body goals $Q_1^{(i)} \wedge \cdots \wedge Q_{k_i}^{(i)}$ $(i = 1, \cdots, m)$ represent a condition to discriminate a category C_i when S is given. Each goal $Q_j^{(i)}$ consists of the disjunction of goals $R_{1_j}^{(i)}; \cdots; R_{h_j}^{(i)}$ where $R_{h_j}^{(i)}$ represents some predicate that discriminates a category C_i, such as $contain(S, \sigma)$ which is *true* when a sequence S contains a pattern σ.

The semantics of stochastic motifs are given from the viewpoint of the computational learning theory of stochastic rules [12]. A stochastic motif represents a probabilistic mapping from protein sequences to categories. The probabilistic mapping can be regarded as a conditional probability distribution over the categories when a sequence is given, by introducing a probability structure on the sequence–category pairs. See the Yamanishi paper [13] for the formal approach to learning stochastic motifs.

3   MDL Learning

MDL learning extracts good rules from given training data, taking account of the balance between a rule's complexity and its fitness to the training data[12]. The most important point is that it enables us to avoid overfitting when extracting stochastic motifs and to extract stable stochastic motifs. In addition, it is useful for improving the convergence performance of genetic algorithms since it gives effective bias for reflecting the complexity of the rules for the fitness function which has a plateau around the optimal solution. The details are discussed in section 6.

The overfitting problem in motif extraction results from noise in protein sequences. The noise arises for various reasons. First is the intrinsic nature of creatures, that is, mutation may occur at any position in a protein sequence. There is no reason to believe that training sequences and test sequences are all mutation free. Second, the protein sequences available now are just a very small portion of species in the world. This means that sampling errors may occur when using the current protein sequence database for training sequences. Lastly, classification errors may occur when a category, which is expected to have a unique motif, does not coincide with the training sequences. Therefore, one should notice that the fittest motif to training sequences does not always mean the best motif in motif extraction. For example, as we have shown in the previous section, the pattern "CXXCH" has exceptions in the cytochrome c. It is possible to avoid these exceptions by adding more conjunctions and disjunctions of patterns such as "AAQCH" and "PGTKM". However, care must be taken so that the obtained result does not become too complex and overfit to the training sequences. Therefore, we adopt the MDL principle to extract simple but stable stochastic motifs which may have exceptions rather than precise motifs without exceptions.

The MDL principle originally comes from coding theory in communication. The basic idea is to optimize the number of bits when sending a piece of information, by means of encoding a rule and its exceptions in the piece of information. The MDL principle selects the encoding that minimizes the total bit length of the rule and the exceptions.

The flavor of the MDL principle is the following. Suppose there is a binary string "101110111010". Sending the string requires 12 bits if we do not use any rule. Fewer bits are sufficient if we compress the string using a rule and its exception. In this case, we can represent the string as three repeats of "101*" with exceptions "110" for the 4th bit of each repeat in place of * in the rule. The rule requires $log3^4 = 6.32^1$ bits since we have to choose one of 3^4 4-character rules using a three characters alphabet (i.e. 1,0,*). The exception requires $log2^3 = 3.0$ bits. The total becomes 9.32 bits. We may find a more complex rule to reduce the number of exceptions, but such a rule might require a longer bit length. Therefore, it is important to balance the complexity of the rule and the number of exceptions to reduce the total bit length.

In our methodology, we apply the MDL principle for extracting stochastic motifs in the way proposed by Yamanishi[12] for learning stochastic rules. In Yamanishi's MDL learning algorithm, the MDL principle selects a stochastic rule that balances the complexity of the stochastic rule and its likelihood of fitness to the training data. The rest of this section follows his algorithm with slight modifications which mainly come from a difference in stochastic rule representation; that is, stochastic decision lists and stochastic decision predicates.

Our methodology selects a stochastic motif that balances the complexity of representation and its fitness for the training sequences. The complexity of a stochastic motif is measured in terms of the description length needed for encoding the probability parameters and the Horn clauses of a stochastic decision predicate. The fitness of a stochastic motif is measured in terms

---

[1] "log" denotes logarithm with base 2.

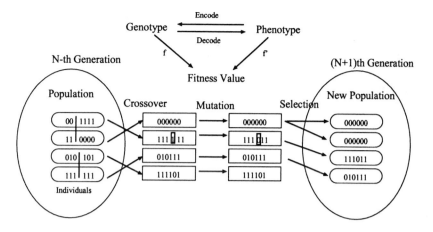

FIG. 3. *Mechanism of Simple Genetic Algorithms*

of the description length of the data relative to the motif, calculated as the negative logarithm of the likelihood of categories for the given motif. The calculation of likelihood and motif complexity is summarized in the appendix.

4 Genetic Algorithms

Genetic algorithms are stochastic search algorithms based on an analogy to biological evolution[3]. As in figure 3, genetic algorithms simulate the survival of the fittest in a population of individuals represented by binary strings. A function, often called a *fitness function*, gives values to the binary strings. The aim of a genetic algorithm is to find a global optimum of the fitness function when given an initial population of individuals by applying genetic operators in each generation. The genetic operators consist of the following: crossover, mutation and selection.

Crossover The crossover operator produces two descendants by exchanging parts of two individuals. This operator aims to produce a better individual by replacing a part of an individual with a better part of another individual. For example, crossover of the strings "000110" and "110111" between the third and fourth bits (referred as third position) produces the strings "000111" and "110110". The candidates for the crossover operation and the crossover position are randomly chosen.

Mutation The mutation operator changes certain bit(s) in an individual. For example, the string "000110" becomes "001110" if mutation occurs at the third bit. This operation aims to keep diversity in a population.

Selection   The selection operator chooses good individuals in a population according to their fitness values and the given selection strategy. This operator aims to increase the numbers of better individuals in the population while maintaining diversity. It simulates the *survival–of–the–fittest* principle. The operator first calculates the relative fitness of all individuals. Then, several lesser individuals are discarded and the same number of better individuals are duplicated according to their relative fitness values. In the case of roulette wheel selection strategy, it selects the next individuals with the probabilities in proportion to their relative fitness values. So, the better an individual the higher its chance of remaining or being duplicated.

One interesting characteristic of our genetic algorithm is its use of the MDL principle to calculate the fitness value of an individual motif. The MDL length gives the natural relative fitness values in the population; the smaller the better in this case. In addition, an asynchronous parallel genetic algorithm is adopted to make use of parallel machines. In this algorithm, the population is divided into a set of subpopulations in which individuals migrate asynchronously.

5   The Experimental Motif Extraction System

The overview of our experimental motif extraction system is the following. The target hypothesis space is the domain of stochastic decision predicates. The search strategy is based on the MDL principle. The search algorithm is an asynchronous parallel genetic algorithm which consists of a set of subpopulations in which individuals migrate asynchronously. In each subpopulation, individuals represent stochastic decision predicates in the target hypothesis space, and the fitness function calculates the corresponding description lengths of the stochastic decision predicates.

5.1   Hypothesis space

The search time depends considerably on the size of the hypothesis space. A too–large hypothesis space makes it difficult for us to find the optimal stochastic decision predicate in a reasonable time. Therefore, as the first step of motif extraction, we restrict the stochastic predicates to the following forms.

```
motif(S,proteinClass) with p1
     :- contain(S,pattern1) and
        contain(S,pattern2) ...
motif(S,others) with p2.
```

That is, we use a predicate *motif* that discriminates the target protein category *proteinClass* from other proteins (*others*) in the database. The discrimination conditions are represented by the conjunction of *contain* predicates. As the pattern candidates in the *contain* predicates, we adopt

128 patterns (or 1024 patterns if needed) that occur frequently in the target proteins.

In the case of ordinal motif representation, the distance between patterns, disjunction of patterns and negative patterns are used as well as the conjunction of patterns. Although it is possible to incorporate these facilities in stochastic decision predicates, the current motif extraction system does not adopt them for the following reasons.

Length Information Some motif representations can specify the minimum and maximum distances between patterns. This distance information is sometimes useful for expressing global motifs that have a redundant region between patterns. However, it is not so easy to estimate the minimum and maximum distances since the protein sequence length can be unexpectedly varied by means of "insertion" and "deletion". In this sense, it would be better to estimate distance distribution rather than to specify maximum and minimum distances, although the method requires more training sequences for precise estimation.

Disjunction Disjunction is an important representation to express varieties of genetic information. Stochastic decision predicates provide two ways to do this; disjunction between clauses and disjunction in a clause. Clause–level disjunction is useful for dividing a category into disjoint subcategories. For example, cytochrome c can be divided into two subcategories; Euglena cytochrome c which has a pattern "AAQCH" and other cytochrome c which has a pattern "CXXCH". To extract clause–level disjunction, the following procedure is effective; first, find a (conjunction of) pattern that mostly distinguishes a target category, then eliminate sequences which have the pattern from training sequences. Iterate the above procedure on the remaining training sequences until sufficient discrimination performance is achieved. In general, the larger the number of clauses, the more discrimination performance is achieved, but the higher the chance of overfitting to the training sequences. The MDL principle may help by balancing the number of clauses and the discrimination performance.

On the other hand, as for disjunctive patterns in a clause, one should consider biological interpretations as well as discrimination performance. A disjunction of patterns corresponding to different sites does not make sense as a motif, even if the disjunction contributes to discrimination performance improvement. The patterns should correspond to the same site. This can be done by multiple alignment of homologous protein sequences or homologous peptide sequences. However, according to our experience, a disjunction of patterns usually consists of one dominant pattern and various subpatterns which is difficult to interpret as a rule. In some sense, this suggests the limitation of stochastic decision predicates in motif representation.

Negative Expression Negative expressions are sometimes useful for representing motifs more precisely. For example, Prosite[2] represents the Cytochrome c motif as "C-{CPWHF}-{CPWR}-C-H-{CFYW}" where {} represents amino acids which *cannot* be at the position. However, it is not appropriate to determine the occurrence of an amino acid so strictly. Actually, some amino acids tends to occur in some positions of the cytochrome c sequence but not with 100 percent certainty. Therefore it would be better to use statistical information at each position in the protein sequences. In addition, the statistical information may take account of the affinity of neighboring amino acids. An HMM representation of stochastic motifs described in section 6 is one such approach.

5.2   Mapping to binary strings

The mapping from a stochastic decision predicate to an N bit binary string is done as follows: First, select the best N basic patterns which frequently occur in the target sequences. In our experience, we used the basic patterns that specify three positions out of three–senven amino acids, such as "AAA", "AAXA" and "AXXXXAA" where X denotes a variable. Then, map the N patterns to each bit of the string so that a bit 1 and 0 represent the occurrence and absense of the pattern in a discrimination condition, respectively. According to this mapping, N bit binary strings can express 2^N kinds of stochastic decision predicates.

For example, suppose we use 3-bit length binary strings whose first, second, third bits correspond to the patterns "CXXCH", "PXLXG", "GXKM", respectively. Then, the binary string "100" represents the following stochastic decision predicate.

```
motif(S,proteinClass) with p1
    :- contain(S,"CXXCH").
motif(S,others) with p2.
```

The binary string "011" represents the following stochastic decision predicate.

```
motif(S,proteinClass) with p1
    :- contain(S,"PXLXG") & contain(S,"GXKM").
motif(S,others) with p2.
```

As for the genetic operators, we adopt one-point crossover, one-point mutation and roulette wheel selection as described in section 4. The values of other runtime parameters are: the adjustment parameter is 1.0, the number of subpopulations is 63, the subpopulation size is 16, the crossover rate is 1.0, the mutation rate is 0.01 and the migration rate is 0.5, that is, one individual per two generations on average.

5.3   Calculation of Fitness Value

The experimental stochastic motif extraction system adopts the MDL principle to calculate fitness values of individuals. As described in section 3, MDL learning takes account of a rule's complexity as well as its fitness to training data. However, it is not easy to compare "rule complexity" and "fitness" since they are different measures on different dimensions. To achieve a quantitative comparison between these two measures, the MDL principle unifies them as "description length".

The description length for the rule complexity is given by calculating the minimum length of binary string required for encoding a motif under the condition that the motif can be decoded from the binary string. The full calculation is shown in the appendix. In the case of stochastic motif extraction, the description length encodes the number of predicates, conjunction and disjunction operators, patterns and discrimination categories in clauses.

Minimum encoding is important for eliminating arbitrariness and sometimes useful for expressing the intrinsic complexity of rules. However, from an engineering point of view, the encoding should be designed so that it reflects biological significance. For example, a pattern "CXXCH" consists of 5 characters chosen from an alphabet of 21 kinds of characters (20 amino acids plus variable X). So, $\log 21^5 = 22.0$ bits is enough to encode it. However, such encoding cannot express the difference between patterns with variables and without a variable if the lengths of patterns are the same.

In case of stochastic motif extraction, the description lengths for variables and amino acids are calculated separately so that the longer the pattern, the longer the description length, and the more variables, the shorter the description length, if the lengths of patterns are the same. The description length for variables is the number of bits required to encode pattern length and variable positions that occur in a pattern. The description length for amino acids is the number of bits to encode possible combinations of 20 amino acids. With this encoding scheme, the description lengths of 'CXXCH" and "AAQCH" become 16.3 and 21.6 bits, respectively. The description length of stochastic decision clauses ($el(CL)$) is the sum of the bit lengths required to encode the information above. In case of stochastic motif extraction from protein superfamilies, $el(CL)$ becomes a fairly large value, comparable to the description length of amino acid and variable patterns, about 20 bits for each pattern in a clause.

The description length of a rule also requires a probability length ($el(PL)$) to encode probabilities estimated for each clause. According to the well-known encoding scheme, it is sufficient to encode the logarithm of the square root of the number of data that become *true* at the clause in order to obtain sufficient accuracy[12]. Therefore, if the number of success data is 100 and 10000, the lengths are 3.32 bits and 6.65 bits, respectively. $el(PL)$ is significant if the number of clauses is large.

The description length to denote the fitness of a stochastic motif is calculated by the logarithmic likelihood of the obtained stochastic motif to the training sequences $(el(LL))$. Likelihood is a good measure used for evaluating the fitness of estimate model to training data and is defined as

$$\prod_{i=1}^{m} p_i^{N_i}(1 - p_i)^{N-N_i}$$

where N is the number of examples that make the ith clause *true*, N_i is the number of examples that make the ith clause *true* and belong to the category specified in the motif, and m is the total number of clauses. A logarithmic likelihood denotes the number of bits to encode likelihood and can be decomposed into the sum of entropy function and Kullback-Leibler information divergence (see Appendix for the details). Although the MDL principle takes account of rule complexity, logarithmic likelihood is still a dominant factor of quantitative measure of goodness. In fact, it easily becomes hundreds of bits if a stochastic motif has a lot of negative examples.

The maximum likelihood method uses only likelihood as a quantitative measure. In other words, the maximum likelihood method is a quantitative measure which selects a rule that mostly fits the training data. Since the dominant factor of the MDL principle is logarithmic likelihood, the optimal rule selected by the MDL principle would converge to the optimal rule selected by the maximum likelihood method if the training data set becomes large enough. The difference appears when training data are quite a few. The MDL principle compensates for the lack of reliability of training data, by the complexities of estimated rules.

An adjustment parameter (λ) is another important factor in this calculation. It gives a weight for rule complexity compared to logarithmic likelihood in order to calculate the total description length of stochastic motif $(el(DL))$. In some sense, it is possible to say that the maximum likelihood method is a special case of the MDL principle, when the adjustment parameter is 0. In the case of our stochastic motif extraction, the adjustment parameter is 1. The effects of the adjustment parameter are discussed in section 6.

6   Discussion

6.1   Experimental Results of Stochastic Motif Extraction

Table 1 contains some of the stochastic motifs extracted by our experimental system when applied to the 166 protein categories that have more than 10 entries in the Protein Identification Resources (PIR32.0) database, which has 2802 superfamilies and 9633 entries[2]. The proteins in the table are the

---

[2] Annotated and classified entries by homology in pirl.dat.

TABLE 1

A portion of stochastic motif extraction

Protein category				Stochastic motif					
$\ell(DL)($	$\ell(CL),$	$\ell(PL),$	$\ell(LL))$	E	$N_1^+,$	N_1	$N_2^+,$	N_2	
Cytochrome-c				CXXCH					
309.544(	18.288,	10.564,	280.693)	140	137,	244	9386,	9389	
Cytochrome p450				FXXGXXXC&CXGXXXA					
95.705(	40.868,	9.179,	45.658)	33	31,	35	9596,	9598	
Trypsin				GWG&CXXDXG					
124.490(	34.253,	9.435,	80.802)	40	37,	50	9580,	9583	
Pepsin				FXXXFD& VPXXXC					
80.802(	38.575,	8.700,	33.526)	19	17,	18	9613,	9615	
Immunoglobulin V region				DXXXYXC					
692.147(	20.095,	10.871,	661.181)	268	237,	379	9223,	9254	
Immunoglobulin C region				CXXXXFXP&FXPXXXXXXW&CLXXXXXP					
289.758(	63.079,	9.477,	217.203)	74	53,	53	9559,	9580	
Globin				PXTXXXF&HGXXV& PXTXXXXXXF					
703.061(	59.915,	10.878,	632.268)	456	382,	383	9176,	9250	

following. *Cytochrome c* is a heme-binding protein that carries an electron in respiratory chain. *Cytochrome p450* is a mono-oxygenase containing a proto-heme. *Trypsin* is a protease secreted from a pancreas. *Pepsin* is an acid protease secreted from the stomach. *Immunoglobulin C region* is a constant region of immunoglobulin C. *Immunoglobulin V region* is a variable region of immunoglobulin C. *Globin* is an apo protein that constructs a hemoglobin when binding with a heme molecule.

In table 1, the column *StochasticMotif* has the conjunctions of patterns extracted by our system. The columns $\ell(DL)$ is the description length of the stochastic motif which is a sum of the description length of the stochastic decision clauses ($\ell(CL)$), the probability length ($\ell(PL)$) and the logarithmic likelihood of the stochastic motif for the training sequences ($\ell(LL)$).

The column E is the number of target protein sequences in the protein sequence database (PIR). The column N_1, N_2 is the number of protein sequences that become *true* at the first and second clauses of the stochastic decision predicate. The column N_1^+, N_2^+ shows the number of protein sequences which belong to the target protein category in N_1 and N_2, respectively.

See the Konagaya paper [7] for the details of stochastic motifs extracted by our system. The correspondence between the obtained stochastic motifs and biologically meaningful regions remains as a future research issue.

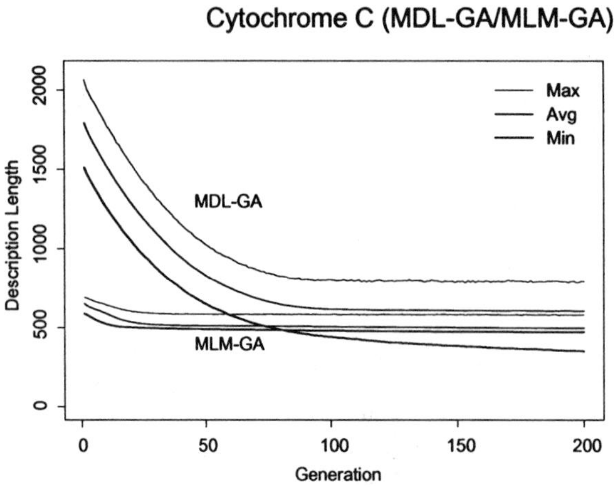

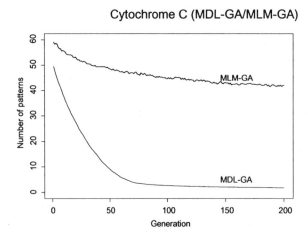

Cytochrome C (MDL-GA/MLM-GA)

FIG. 4. *Average description lengths of the best stochastic motif encountered in each generation*

Cytochrome C (MDL-GA/MLM-GA)

FIG. 5. *Average number of patterns of the best stochastic motif encountered in each generation*

TABLE 2

Prediction error rates (percent) for Cytochrome C by Cross Validation Method

	MDL-GA	MLM-GA
$(\sum_{i=1}^{10} E_i^+)/N^+$	2.1	40.7
$(\sum_{i=1}^{10} E_i^-)/N^-$	1.0	0
$(\sum_{i=1}^{10} E_i^+ + E_i^-)/(N^+ + N^-)$	1.1	0.6

6.2   Comparison of the MDL principle and the Maximum likelihood method

To demonstrate the effectiveness of the MDL principle, various indices including prediction errors and convergence speed are compared to the maximum likelihood method (MLM). In MLM, good individuals are selected using only the description length of likelihood ($\ell(LL)$) without consideration for the complexity of a stochastic decision predicate ($\ell(CL) + \ell(PL)$).

Using a cross validation technique, the prediction errors can be counted as follows. Let S_i be a disjoint subgroup of protein sequences S for certain N where $S = \cup_{i=1}^{N} S_i$. Let S_i' be a training set which removes the i th subgroup from the original protein sequences ($S_i' = S - S_i$). Then, let M_i be a stochastic motif extracted from the training set S_i', and count the number of prediction errors E_i^+ and E_i^- using the subgroup S_i as a test set. E_i^+ shows the number of protein sequences that belong to the target protein category but are not *true* for the first clause of the stochastic motif M_i, and E_i^- shows the number of protein sequences that do not belong to the target protein category but are *true* for the first clause of the stochastic motif M_i.

Table 2 shows the prediction errors for cytochrome c by the cross validation method when the test set is divided into 10 subgroups, each of which saves in turn as the training set for the remaining nine subgroups. The best scored stochastic motif is selected from 50 trials for each subgroup. Each trial requires 200 genetic algorithm generations.

The results show that the stochastic motifs obtained using a genetic algorithm with the MDL principle (MDL-GA) are more stable than the ones obtained using a genetic algorithm with the maximum likelihood method (MLM-GA). As seen in table 2, the stochastic motifs obtained by MLM-GA are apparently overfitted to the sample protein sequences. MLM-GA shows strong discrimination performance for the sample protein sequences ($\sum_{i=1}^{10} E_i^-$), but shows weak predictive performance for the test sequences ($\sum_{i=1}^{10} E_i^+$).

Contrary to our expectations, the result does not comes from the intrinsic difference between MDL and MLM, but comes from the difference of convergence speeds between MDL-GA and MLM-GA. As shown in figure 4, MDL-GA shows good convergence speed compared to MLM-GA. That is, MLM-GA is too slow to give us the global optimum in the search space

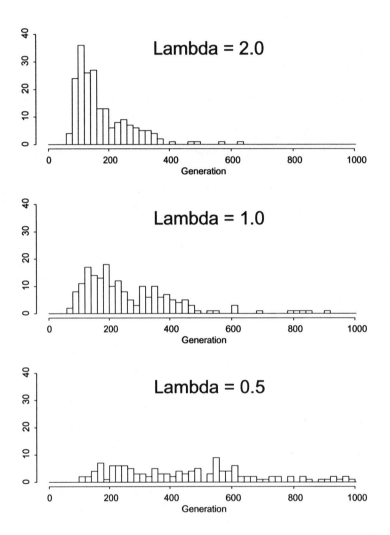

FIG. 6. *Comparison of convergence speeds by the distributions of generations in which the optimal solution is found*

TABLE 3

The number of times optimal solution is not found (in 100 trials)

Mutation Rate	0.005	0.01	0.015	0.02–0.03
Sequential GA	2	0	0	0
Parallel GA	10	3	1	0

within a reasonable time. The difference in the convergence speeds comes from the bias caused by the MDL principle. As shown in figure 5, MDL-GA rapidly decreases the number of patterns in the best stochastic motif encountered, while MLM-GA gradually decreases. This is natural since the description length of Horn clauses basically corresponds to the number of patterns. In other words, the MDL principle biases GA to select individuals with fewer patterns.

Figure 6 shows the effect of the bias on the convergence speed of a genetic algorithm with the MDL principle as the adjustment parameter (λ) changes from 0.5 to 2.0. The histogram in figure 6 shows the distribution of generations in which the optimal solution (CXXCH) is found. In case of $\lambda = 0.0$, that is, the genetic algorithm with the maximum likelihood method, no optimum stochastic motif is found as far as we have tried (10000 generations, 10000 trials).

6.3   Parallel Genetic Algorithm

One of the advantages of genetic algorithms is the potential for performance speed up using parallelism. To make use of parallel machines, we adopt an asynchronous parallel genetic algorithm. In this algorithm, the population is divided into sets of subpopulations in which individuals migrate asynchronously. The migration overhead is negligible and 7.7 times speedup is observed when using 8 processors on a shared memory machine.

According to our experience whith stochastic motif extraction, the following phenomena have been observed in terms of the parallelism of genetic algorithms. As seen in figure 7, parallel GA is slightly better than sequential GA with respect to the average generation in which the optimal solution is found, if the total number of individuals are the same. The average generation varies according to mutation rates and has an optimal rate around 0.01 when the total number of individuals is 128 and the number of subgroups is 8. However, we also observed that the smaller the mutation rate, the higher the chance of missing an optimal solution (see table 3). This result supports the theory that a small mutation rate cannot keep sufficient diversity in a population and tends to cause early convergence especially when the population is small. In addition, it should be noted that the communication overhead between processing elements is almost negligible if asynchronous migration facility is provided.

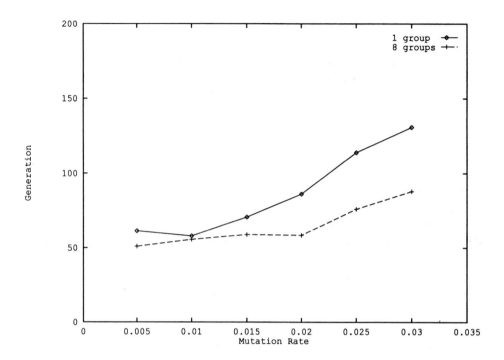

FIG. 7. *Comparison of sequential GA and parallel GA*

6.4 Stochastic Motif by HMM

Stochastic motif extraction using stochastic decision predicates has success-
fully extracted stable stochastic motifs from protein sequences. However, the
decision predicates are sometimes too simple to represent stochastic motifs
and suffer from relatively low prediction accuracy due to strict symbolic
pattern matching, the lack of constraint facilities on variables, the restricted
usage of statistical information on neighbor amino acids, and so on. In order
to achieve higher discrimination accuracy, we have studied hidden Markov
models (HMM) as an alternative representation of stochastic motifs. Figure 8 shows an example of an HMM corresponding to the cytochrome c
motif "CXXCH". As seen in the figure, HMM can express statistical information about amino acids occurring at the variables (X) in the symbolic
pattern "CXXCH" by means of observation probabilities of observed symbols (amino acids in this case) and transition probabilities from node to
node. The statistical information not only improves prediction accuracy
but also gives intuitive interpretation of stochastic motifs. For example, it
is possible to say that smaller amino acids frequently occur at the second
and third nodes in the cytochrome c motif. In addition, it should be noted
that HMM can handle disjunctive patterns and exceptional patterns naturally. For example, the HMM in figure 8 does not recognize "A" at the first

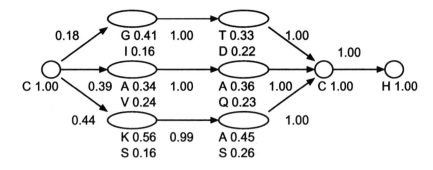

FIG. 8. *HMM representation of cytochrome c motif (CXXCH)*

node[3] but the entire HMM can discriminate "AAQCH" as a cytochrome c motif.

7 Conclusion

Knowledge discovery in genetic sequences is demonstrated using stochastic motif extraction as an example. Our methodology is characterized by the stochastic representation of motifs using stochastic decision predicates, quantitative criteria using the MDL principle and fast search algorithms using genetic algorithms. Our experimental results show that the methodology actually produces stable motifs from real protein sequences. The effectiveness of GA with the MDL principle has been statistically proven and compared to GA with the maximum likelihood method, although data are limited to cytochrome c. The effectiveness of parallel genetic algorithms and the HMM representation of stochastic motifs were also noted. We believe the methodology can also be applied to the various kind of knowledge discovery in genetic sequences.

Acknowledgements

Most of this research has been done in the Fifth Generation Computer Systems Research Project promoted by MITI. The author wishes to express his sincere gratitude to Dr. K. Nitta of ICOT for his encouragement and support. The author also thanks Dr. K. Yamanishi for his technical advice especially for the MDL principle, Mr. S. Oyanagi of NSIS for his cooperation on collecting the data required for this research and the genetic information group between ICOT and NEC Corporation for their valuable discussion and advice.

---

[3]In actual, the observation probability for "A" is not 0 but a very small number.

References

[1] Aitken, Alastair, *Identification of Protein Consensus Sequences*, Ellis Horwood Series in Biochemistry and Biotechnology, (1990).

[2] Bairoch,A, *PROSITE: A Dictionary of Protein Sites and Patterns*, User's Manual, (1991).

[3] Goldberg,D.E., *Genetic Algorithms in Search, Optimization, and Machine Learning*, Addison-Wesley Publishing Company, Inc.,(1989).

[4] Fujiwara,Y. and Konagaya, A., *Protein Motif Extraction using a Hidden Markov Model*, Proc. of Genome Informatics Workshop IV, Tokyo, (1993),pp.56-64.

[5] Konagaya, A., and Yamanishi,K.: *A Stochastic Decision Predicate: A Scheme to Represent Motifs*, The AAAI Workshop of Classification and Pattern Recognition in Molecular Biology, (1991).

[6] Konagaya, A., *A Stochastic Approach to Genetic Information Processing*, The Workshop on Algorithmic Learning Theory ALT'92,(1992).

[7] Konagaya, A. and Kondo, Y., *Stochastic Motif Extraction using a Genetic Algorithm with the MDL Principle*, in Hawaii Int. Conf. on System Sciences, (1993).

[8] Rissanen, J., *Modeling by shortest data description*, Automatica, 14 (1978), pp.465-471.

[9] Rooman,M.J. and Wodak,S.J., *Identification of Predictive Sequence Motifs limited by Protein Structure Data Base Size*, Nature, vol.335, 1 (1988), pp.45-49.

[10] Shimozono,S, Shinohara,A., Shinohara,T., Miyano,S., Kuhara,S. and Arikawa,S., *An Approach to Bioinformatical Knowledge Acquisition*, in Hawaii International Conference on System Sciences, (1993).

[11] Smith,H.O., Annau,T.M. and Chandrasegaran, S., *Finding Sequence Motifs in Groups of Functionally Related Proteins*, in Proc. Natl. Acad. Sci. USA, vol.87, (1990), pp.826-830.

[12] Yamanishi, K.: *A learning criterion for stochastic rules*, Proceedings of the 3-rd Annual Workshop on Computational Learning Theory, Morgan Kaufmann, (1990), pp. 67-81.

[13] Yamanishi, K. & Konagaya, A., Leaning Stochastic Motifs from Genetic Sequences. *in Proc. of the Eighth International Workshop of Machine Learning*,(1991).

[14] Rissanen, J., A universal prior for integers and estimation by minimum description length. *Annals of Statistics, 11,*(1983), 416-431.

Appendix: How to calculate the description length of stochastic motifs

Description Length of Likelihood   Let $\ell(LL)$ be the logarithmic likelihood of a stochastic motif for a set of training sequences. The likelihood of the stochastic motif can be calculated using probabilities associated for categories on each Horn clause in the stochastic motif.

Let $(S_1, C_1), \cdots, (S_N, C_N)$ be N training sequence and category pairs. Let E_j be the set of sequences which are **false** for the $1, \cdots, j - 1$th clauses and **true** for the jth clause. Let N_j be the number of sequences in E_j and let N_j^+ be the number of sequences which are in E_j and belong to the category of the j-th clause. Then the likelihood of the categories $(C_1, \cdots, C_N)$ when given training sequences $(S_1, \cdots, S_N)$ with respect to a stochastic predicate with probabilities $(p_1, \cdots, p_m)$, which we denote LL, is calculated as follows.

$$LL = \prod_{j=1}^{m} p_j^{N_j^+} (1 - p_j)^{N_j - N_j^+}.$$

The description length $\ell(LL)$ is given by $-\log LL$ which can be calculated, as follows:

$$(1) \qquad \ell(LL) = \sum_{i=1}^{m} N_i \{ H(\tilde{p}_i) + D_{KL}(\tilde{p}_i \parallel \hat{p}_i) \}$$

where $\tilde{p}_i = N_i^+/N_i$ and $\hat{p}_i$ is an estimate of the true parameter p_i^*, which is set to be $\frac{N_i^+ + 1}{N_i + 2}$ (the Bayes estimator) to avoid the difficulties of calculating the description length when $N_i^+ = 0$ or N_i. In addition, $H(\tilde{p}_i)$ and $D_{KL}(\tilde{p}_i \parallel \hat{p}_i)$ are the entropy function and Kullback-Leibler divergence defined as follows.

$$H(\tilde{p}_i) = -\tilde{p}_i \log \tilde{p}_i - (1 - \tilde{p}_i) \log(1 - \tilde{p}_i)$$

$$D_{KL}(\tilde{p}_i \parallel \hat{p}_i) = \tilde{p}_i \log \frac{\tilde{p}_i}{\hat{p}_i} + (1 - \tilde{p}_i) \log \frac{1 - \tilde{p}_i}{1 - \hat{p}_i}$$

The description length $\ell(LL)$ indicates the number of bits required to encode the distribution of positive examples and negative examples relative to the stochastic decision predicate. The length varies from near 0 bit[4], when $p_i = 0$ or 1.0 $(i = 1, \cdots, m)$, to N bits, when $p_i = 0.5 (i = 1, \cdots, m)$. The former occurs when the stochastic decision predicate completely discriminates the target categories in the given sequences. The latter occurs when the stochastic decision predicate does not contribute to any discrimination of the given sequences.

Description Length of Probabilities   Let $\ell(PL)$ be the description length of the probabilities $\hat{P} = (\hat{p}_1, \cdots \hat{p}_m)$ for a stochastic decision predicate. Since the accuracy (variance) of the maximum likelihood estimator is $O(1/\sqrt{N})$, the description length $\ell(PL)$ is given by:

$$(2) \qquad \ell(PL) = \sum_{i=1}^{m} \frac{\log N_i}{2}$$

---

[4]It is not appropriate to neglect the value of Kullback-Leibler divergence when the value of entropy function is small.

Description Length of Horn Clauses   Let $\ell(CL)$ be the description length of the Horn clauses CL. $\ell(CL)$ significantly depends on the encoding scheme from Horn clauses to binary strings. The scheme ought to be designed so that the description length can reflect the complexity of the Horn clauses.

In the motif extraction system, $\ell(CL)$ is given by:

$$
\begin{aligned}
\ell(CL) \;=\; & \sum_{i=1}^{m} \Big[\, \log^*\Big(\sum_{j=1}^{k_i} h_j\Big) + \Big(\sum_{j=1}^{k_i} h_j - 1\Big) \\
& + \sum_{j=1}^{k_i}\sum_{l=1}^{h_j}\Big\{\log\binom{L_l^j(i)}{X_l^j(i)} \\
& + (L_l^j(i) - X_l^j(i))*\log(|\,\mathcal{A}\,|)\Big\} + \log r\,\Big]
\end{aligned}
$$

(3)

where $L_l^j(i)$ and $X_l^j(i)$ are the number of amino acids and of variables, respectively, in the pattern in the l–th predicate in the j–th disjunction region of the i–th clause. On the righthand of (3), the first term denotes the description length of the number of *contain* predicates in the i–th clause. For any $d > 0$, $\log^* d$ denotes $\log d + \log\log d + \cdots$ where the sum is taken over all positive terms (Rissanen's integer coding scheme [14]). The second term of (3) denotes the description length to encode the disjunctions and conjunctions occurring in the i–th clause. The third term denotes the description length of the positions of variables in the pattern σ appearing in the predicate '$contain(S,\sigma)$.' The fourth term denotes the description length required to describe amino acids (not variables) included in the pattern σ appearing in the predicate '$contain(S,\sigma)$'. $|\,\mathcal{A}\,|$ is the cardinality of amino acid set $\mathcal{A}$; 20 in this case. The last term $\log r$ denotes the description length of the category C appearing in the predicate '$motif(S,C)$'.

Description Length of Stochastic Motif   By summing (1), (2), and (3), we have the following description length $\ell(DL)$ of a stochastic motif represented by a decision predicate:

(4)
$$
\begin{aligned}
&\ell(DL)\\
&\stackrel{\text{def}}{=} \ell(LL) + \lambda\{\ell(PL) + \ell(CL)\}
\end{aligned}
$$

where λ is the adjustment parameter. The MDL principle asserts that one should select the stochastic motif which minimizes the description length $\ell(DL)$.

Chapter 8
Bandwidth, Granularity, and Mechanisms: Key Issues in the Design of Parallel Computers

William J. Dally[1]

Abstract

Parallel computer design involves trading off ease of programming against cost and performance. While the programmer would like a flat address space with equal bandwidth to all locations, most of the cost/performance advantage of a parallel computer comes from providing a bandwidth hierarchy. While the programmer would like to have a single powerful processor, the best performance and cost/performance is achieved with many smaller processors. A machine designer must achieve a balance between these conflicting demands. Designing appropriate mechanisms to expose relevant aspects of the machine to the programmer while minimizing overhead and hiding arcane features is also central to a successful machine design. This paper addresses these issues drawing examples from the J-Machine and M-Machine projects at MIT as well as from some recent commercial parallel computers.

1. Introduction

Parallel computers today are used primarily in specialized, high-end applications. Trends in integrated-circuit technology, however, promise to make parallel computers pervasive. The density of integrated circuit chips is increasing at a much faster rate than their speed. Parallelism converts this increased density into performance. Today, a fully-pipelined superscalar microprocessor fits comfortably on a single chip along with a cache memory. Such processors exploit instruction-level parallelism through pipelining and multiple-issue. Further increases in circuit density will demand a more explicit approach to parallelism. A challenge to the designer is to provide an incremental path for users to migrate from sequential to explicitly parallel computers.

---

[1] Artificial Intelligence Laboratory and Laboratory for Computer Science, Massachusetts Institute of Technology, 545 Technology Square, Cambridge, MA 02139, billd@ai.mit.edu

A parallel machine designer is faced with three major issues:

Bandwidth: How should the bandwidth of the system vary from local connections (e.g., registers to ALU) to global connections (e.g., global memory access)? Cost factors motivate a reduction in bandwidth from local to global. Local bandwidth is cheap while global bandwidth is expensive. A balance must be struck, however, for if global bandwidth is reduced too far, the machine becomes difficult to program and its application space becomes limited as there is only so much locality in typical applications.

Resource Distribution: There are two aspects to this issue: how should the machine be divided into nodes (granularity), and how should the cost of each node be divided between processor, memory, and communication (balance). The granularity issue is driven by memory capacity. The best cost/performance is realized at the smallest granularity that provides adequate memory bandwidth. Balance within a node is achieved when the incremental performance gain realized by an incremental increase in cost is the same for each component of the machine.

Mechanisms: To convert parallelism to performance, control overhead must be reduced by providing efficient yet flexible mechanisms for communication and synchronization. Communication mechanisms, such as a SEND instruction and a receive thread, allow a processor to perform an arbitrary action on a remote node in time comparable to the network latency. To synchronize with events, a processor must be agile, able to switch tasks quickly when waiting on an event.

The remainder of this paper discusses these issues in more detail. We start in Section 2 by examining the constraints that drive parallel computer design, both cultural and technical. Bandwidth is treated in Section 3 by traversing the M-Machine bandwidth hierarchy with a discussion of bandwidth and cost at each stage. Section 4 deals with granularity and balance. Mechanisms are described in Section 5.

2. Constraints

Parallel computer design is constrained by the circuit technology used to build the machine, the characteristics of the applications the computer is intended to run, and the culture of the intended user community. This section examines these issues to constrain the search space for design variables.

2.1 Users require an evolutionary path to parallelism.

The vast majority of computer application programs today are sequential . Enterprises that use computation in the course of their business rely heavily on sequential computers running sequential programs.   Very often, these sequential programs have been evolved over many years at considerable cost to provide an effective solution to the user's problem. The typical user is attracted to the cost/performance advantages of parallel computers, but is unwilling to give up their software legacy to take advantage of parallelism. To satisfy such users, a parallel computer must run sequential codes unchanged and provide an incremental path to parallelism. Once an application has migrated to a parallel platform, it can be modified incrementally to exploit parallelism.

The typical computer system runs many applications.   Those that are compute bound, time-critical applications are good candidates for parallelization.   Many others would not benefit from parallelization because they are not computationally demanding and/or not run frequently. The utility of the computer system, however, depends on being able to run all of these applications.   Often to do this the parallel computer must provide binary API compatibility with some serial architecture for which shrink wrap applications are available.

A third reason for incremental parallelism is the culture of applications programmers.   Most programmers are skilled in writing sequential programs and have little knowledge of parallel programming.   They are comfortable writing sequential programs in sequential programming languages.   It is easier for this cadre of programmers to parallelize sequential programs using extensions to a sequential language than to write a new program from scratch in some inherently parallel programming notation.

The need for an incremental path for parallelism places one constraint on the design of a parallel computer system: A parallel computer must be a good sequential computer, competitive with the best available sequential computers of the day.   It is unacceptable to sacrifice sequential performance for the sake of parallelism. This constraint most strongly affects the design of the memory system for a parallel computer. To compete with a sequential computer with the same total amount of memory, a parallel computer must be able to run a program on a single node that can access any memory location in the machine with latency comparable to that of a sequential computer.

2.2 Each generation, chips get a lot denser and a little faster.

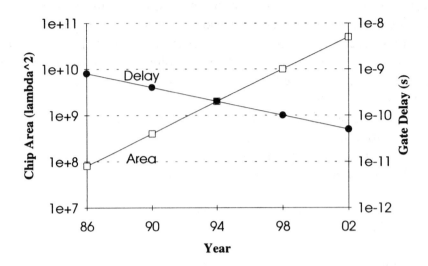

Figure 1: Trends in integrated circuit technology. Chip area is increasing at a rate of 50% per year while gate delay is improving at 20% per year.

Figure 1 shows recent trends in integrated circuit technology extrapolated forward eight years. The figure shows that chip area (in λ^2) is increasing at 50% per year while gate delay is decreasing by 20% per year [HJ91]. Area is expressed in units (λ^2) scaled to the line width of the technology; λ is half a drawn gate length [MC78]. In units of λ^2 the area of a given function, e.g., a bit of SRAM or a 64-bit adder, remains approximately constant across several generations of technology. The area increase is due to improvements in both feature size and chip area. Every four years, the linear feature sizes of a process, e.g., metal pitch and drawn gate length, are reduced by a factor of two. During the same period the chip area that can be manufactured at a fixed yield is increased by 30%. In combination, these two effects give a factor of five improvement in area (in λ^2) every four years.

The gate delay line in Figure 1 shows the delay of a CMOS inverter driving four identical inverters as a function of time. While this delay is a function of many parameters (gate oxide thickness, effective gate length, and parasitics) to first order it is proportional to the linear feature size of the process. With constant field scaling of voltage with feature size, the time required for an electron to cross from one side of a channel to the other (the transit time, τ) is directly proportional to the gate length. Thus, to first order, a 1998 0.3μ (gate length) process can be expected to have half the gate delay (100ps) of a 1994 0.6μ process (200ps). A typical clock cycle is 30-50 gate delays or 100-160MHz for the '94 process and

200-330MHz for the '98 process. While available area has increased by a factor of five, operating speed has increased only by a factor of two.

To put the scaling of chip area in perspective, Table 1 shows the area of some common computer building blocks. The table shows that a powerful sequential processor (without cache or TLB) can be built in about $300M\lambda^2$ of chip area. The 16KByte (128Kbit) cache typically associated with such a processor takes another $200M\lambda^2$ for a total chip area of $500M\lambda^2$. Figure 1 shows that chips of this area became feasible in 1991. Before this time, one either had to use several chips to build a powerful sequential processor or trade area for reduced performance, for example by using an unpipelined floating-point unit. Beyond this point, a designer is challenged by the abundance of chip area. A 2002 chip with $50G\lambda^2$ will be capable of holding 100 such high-performance sequential processors that will operate at close to 8 times the speed of the '91 processor.

Unit	Area (λ^2)
1 bit SRAM	1.5×10^3
P-port register bit	$8(5+P)^2$
4-port register bit	5×10^3
64-bit integer ALU	2×10^6
64-bit pipelined floating-point unit	2×10^8
64-bit processor with FPU	3×10^8

Table 1: Area of some common computer building blocks.

During the 1980s, the performance of single chip microprocessors increased at a rate of about 50% per year. This performance increase had little to do with the switch to simpler RISC instruction sets as evidenced by the corresponding increase in the performance of complex instruction set computer families such as the Intel x86. During this period processors were able to convert increasing chip area to increasing performance by incorporating more features of multi-chip "mainframe" computers. Some of these features, e.g., multiple execution units, involve modest amounts of programmer-invisible parallelism.

By 1991, microprocessors had caught up with mainframes. Beyond this point, converting increases in chip area to performance requires more aggressive use of parallelism. For the next few years, designers will add multiple parallel execution paths under the control of a single sequential program. Such "superscalar" processors are limited to roughly 4-fold parallelism by the amount of instruction-level parallelism available in non-vector sequential programs and the complexity of the instruction issue logic. Explicit parallelism is required to move beyond these limits of instruction-level parallelism.

Trends in integrated circuit technology constitute a parallel imperative for the computer designer. Unless parallelism is used to convert the rapid increase in circuit density to performance, computer performance will only increase with circuit speed, at about 20% per year.

3. Bandwidth

As chip densities and clock frequencies increase, bandwidth becomes the limiting factor to system cost and performance. Improvements in circuit technology have made processors and memory faster and less expensive resulting in an increasingly difficult communication problem. The packaging technology used to interconnect chips into systems is improving at a slower rate than the circuits, and signals are constrained to propagate at a fraction of the speed of light. To achieve good cost/performance, parallel processors must exploit locality to use bandwidth on-chip where it is cheap and minimize demands on global bandwidth which is expensive.

A key decision in the design of a parallel computer is how best to taper bandwidth from its peak at the processor's ALUs to its minimum at the far reaches of the system. If bandwidth is kept too flat between these two points the system will be prohibitively expensive as evidenced by contemporary parallel vector processors such as the Cray YMP-C90. If the bandwidth drops off too fast, the machine will be difficult to program and/or support only a limited class of operations. This is the case with many contemporary massively parallel processors that have bandwidth ratios in excess of 10^3:1. Between these two extremes, a modest bandwidth taper gives good performance on a wide range of applications at minimum cost.

Table 2 shows the bandwidth at each level of the MIT M-Machine [KD92]. Each node contains 12 64-bit (8-Byte) ALUs that operate at 100MHz. The connection between these ALUs and their register files has a bandwidth of 29GBytes/s per node. For a system of 256 nodes, the total register bandwidth is 7.4TBytes/s. At this lowest level of the system, the bandwidth is nearly free as the connections between the ALUs and their co-located register files are very short, about 1mm, and entirely on chip. Thus these connections cost little chip area and zero chip or connector pins.

Location	BW (each)	Per Node	BW (Node)	BW (System)	Ratio
ALU/Register	2.4×10^9	12	2.9×10^{10}	7.4×10^{12}	144
Inter-Register file	8.0×10^8	4	3.2×10^9	8.2×10^{11}	16
Cache	8.0×10^8	4	3.2×10^9	8.2×10^{11}	16
Local Memory	8.0×10^8	1	8.0×10^8	2.0×10^{11}	4
Local Network Channel	8.0×10^8	1	8.0×10^8	2.0×10^{11}	4
Bisection Bandwidth				5.0×10^{10}	1

Table 2: Bandwidth in Bytes/s at each level of the MIT M-Machine.

Table 3 shows the cost of bandwidth at each level of the system. Both cost per Byte/sec and total cost for the system are shown. The table assumes that chip area costs $1\$/10M\lambda^2$ (a $5G\lambda^2$ chip in '96 for $500), package (chip) pins cost $0.20 each, and board pins cost $0.50 each. The package pin cost includes the cost of the package, the board, and assembly and is based on experience from the MIT J-Machine [Da92a]. The board pin cost includes the cost of connectors, cable assemblies, and related mechanical components. The derivations for each row are discussed in the paragraphs below. The table shows that while the bandwidth drops off (by a factor of 144) as one moves from the local to the global levels, the cost of the bandwidth increases more rapidly. The global bandwidth costs more than all of the other components combined. The cost per unit bandwidth varies by a factor of 2500 across the levels of the system.

Location	BW (System)	Area (bit)	Area (chip)	Area (total)	Chip Pins	Board Pins	Cost (B/s)	Cost (sys)
ALU/Register	7.4×10^{12}	$32K\lambda^2$	$74M\lambda^2$	$19G\lambda^2$			2.6×10^{-10}	1900
Inter-Register file	8.2×10^{11}	$480K\lambda^2$	$120M\lambda^2$	$31G\lambda^2$			3.8×10^{-9}	3100
Cache	8.2×10^{11}	$480K\lambda^2$	$120M\lambda^2$	$31G\lambda^2$			3.8×10^{-9}	3100
Local Memory	2.0×10^{11}				128		3.3×10^{-8}	6600
Local Network	2.0×10^{11}				192		4.9×10^{-8}	9800
Bisection	5.0×10^{10}					256	6.6×10^{-7}	33000

Table 3: Cost of bandwidth at each level of the MIT M-Machine.

The M-Machine groups the 12 ALUs into four clusters of 3 ALUs each to exploit locality at the register level. Four inter-cluster buses are used to transfer data between clusters. This 9:1 reduction in bandwidth from the cluster level to the inter-cluster level is motivated by the increasing cost of bandwidth as a function of distance on chip. As indicated in Table 1, the cost of a register bit depends quadratically on the number of ports of a register file. To feed 12 ALUs out of a single register file would require 36 ports giving an area of $110K\lambda^2$ per bit or a prohibitive $5.3G\lambda^2$ for the ~50K register bits in the M-Machine. Most of this area is spent realizing the internal crossbar switch that connects every register to every port. The M-Machine reduces this communication cost by partitioning the registers into 7-port register files ($9.2K\lambda^2$ per bit) for a total register area of 460M λ^2 . The communication between the clusters is factored out into the four buses where these 15mm channels consume $480K\lambda^2$ per bit or $120M\lambda^2$ for the 4 64-bit buses. The cache interface is also implemented as four chip-wide buses and thus has the same cost and performance.

Using synchronous DRAM components, the interface to the local main memory transfers one 64-bit word per 10ns clock. This interface requires about 128 package pins per node which gives the cost shown in Table 3.

The required bandwidth also puts a lower bound on the amount of memory per node if the memory is to be constructed with standard DRAM components. The capacity of DRAM components is growing at about the 50% per year rate shown for chip area in Figure 1. The bandwidth of DRAM components on the other hand is increasing at about 10% per year. The ratio of capacity to bandwidth, the minimum time required to fill or empty the DRAM, is increasing at 40% per year. Current 16Mbit synchronous DRAM components with a bandwidth of 200MBytes/s have a time constant of 10ms. For systems where this constant is larger than the time constant of the applications, the memory is bandwidth rather than capacity limited and the cost per unit bandwidth becomes the cost of the additional memory capacity required to achieve that bandwidth. For 16Mbit DRAMs, this cost is about 5×10^{-7} dollars per MB/s or about 150 times the number shown in the table. This cost of memory bandwidth will play a major role in the discussion of granularity below.

The M-Machine network uses 32-bit wide channels that operate at twice the processor clock and use simultaneous bidirectional signalling [DLD93]. Thus the six channels leaving each node require 192 signal pins. Although there are six channels out of the node, the node is only capable of sending one word per clock into the network. This is the local network bandwidth, the network bandwidth in the absence of contention (or the bandwidth for references to nearby nodes). Four M-Machine nodes are packaged on a multi-chip-module (MCM) and these are cabled to nearby modules to form a 3-D mesh network. For the 256-node machine under consideration, 32 channels cross the bisection of the machine in each direction giving a bisection bandwidth of 64 words per clock, a quarter of the local network and memory bandwidth. Table 3 assigns the cost of the package pins to the local bandwidth and the cost of the MCM-MCM connections to the global bandwidth. While, the two are difficult to separate, any machine providing the same bisection bandwidth will need approximately the same number of board-level connections.

Having the local network bandwidth equal the local memory bandwidth enables the M-Machine to be a good sequential processor. A program can run on a single node and access all the memory in the machine with the same bandwidth that it has to its local DRAM memory. The latency for these remote access is slightly higher than for local references which causes some degradation in sequential performance.

In a 256-node M-Machine, the bandwidth available to access global memory without regard to locality is one quarter of the local memory bandwidth. This arrangement results in a machine that is significantly cheaper than one that provides flat memory bandwidth, a uniform-memory-access or UMA machine. As with cache memories, a bandwidth hierarchy exploits the locality inherent in most applications to realize a significant cost/performance advantage. A machine such as the CM-5 with a local to remote bandwidth ratio of about 100:1 is somewhat less expensive. However, when this bandwidth ratio is this large, the machine becomes much more difficult to program and its application space becomes limited. While the optimum ratio of local to global bandwidth is a subject for research and debate, ratios of 3:1 to 15:1 appear to offer the best compromise between cost/performance and programmability.

The ratio of local memory/network bandwidth to register bandwidth on the M-Machine is 36:1 (12 ALU operations per word of memory bandwidth). Compared to many conventional architectures, this number appears high by a factor of six, and suggests that the M-Machine's ALUs may occasionally become starved for lack of memory bandwidth. This is intentional. Processor utilization, often cited as a measure of utility, is irrelevant. As the tables above show, processors are relatively inexpensive. Memory and network bandwidth are the critical resources in a modern computer system. Inexpensive processors should be added to keep the critical bandwidth resources busy.

4. Granularity and Balance

A key decision in the design of a computer system is the division of resources between processors, memory, and communications [Da92b,YDA94]. One aspect of this decision is granularity: given a fixed budget, should one build many inexpensive processing nodes or a few expensive ones. An any granularity, the designer must also balance the machine by dividing resources between processors, memory, and communications. In Section 3, the division of cost across the bandwidth hierarchy is one example of balance. In this section we will look at the processor-memory balance.

4.1 Balance by cost, not capacity to speed ratio.

In 1967, Amdahl [HP90] suggested that a computer system be balanced by ratio of processor performance (instructions/s or i/s) to memory capacity (Bytes). Specifically, he stated that a system should have 1MByte of memory for each Mi/s of processor performance. The processor performance/size ratio ($i/(s{\times}cm^2)$) benefits from technology improvements in both density (50%/year) and speed (20%/year) while the memory capacity/size ratio (Bytes/cm^2) benefits only from density improvements. Thus the processor to memory cost ratio for an Amdahl-balanced system scales inversely with speed improvements.

Let $K(67)$ denote the ratio of processor cost to memory cost for such an Amdahl-balanced system in 1967. If the processor improves linearly with both area and speed, the capacity of the memory must be increased by 80% per year to maintain the balance at a cost increase of 20% per year. Thus, the processor to memory ratio during year x>67 is given by $K(x)=K(67)1.2^{(67-x)}$. The ratio today would be, $K(94) = .007K(67)$. If we assume $K(67)\sim0.5$, then this projection is consistent with the observation that the ratio of processor to memory area for a modern 64-bit RISC processor $(300M\lambda^2)$ with 64MBytes of DRAM $(50G\lambda^2)$ is less than 1% (0.006).

The cost of a conventional machine has become largely insensitive to processor size as a result of this exponential trend in the ratio of processor to memory size. Thus, processor designers have become lavish in their use of area[2]. Costly features such as large caches, complex data paths, and complex instruction-issue logic are added even though their marginal affect on processor performance (compared to a small cache and a simple organization) is minor. As long as the cost of the machine is dominated by memory, adding area to the processor has a small effect on overall size and cost.

A more economical design results if a machine is balanced based on cost. A machine is *cost-balanced* when the incremental performance increase due to an incremental increase in the cost of each component is equal. Let each component k_i in a machine with performance P have cost c_i, then the machine is cost-balanced if $\partial P/\partial c_i=\partial P/\partial c_j$ $\forall i,j$ [Da86, Da92b].

It is difficult to solve these balance equations because no analytic function exists that relates system performance to component cost and this relationship varies greatly depending on the application being run. Also, analyzing existing applications can be misleading as they have been tuned to run on particular machines and hence reflect the balance of those machines.

Given that memory currently dominates the cost of a computer system, one can approximate cost balance by adding processor resources until they reach some fraction of total cost, for example 10%. Such a system would cost at most 10% more than an Amdahl-balanced system but have 16 times the processor resources. As described above, even if these processors are lightly utilized, providing an excess of processor resources will increase the duty factor on the critical memory and network bandwidth resources.

To make reasonable balancing decisions, it is important to use manufacturing cost, not component price, as our measure of cost. This

---

[2]As a result of this lavish use of area, processor sizes have scaled slightly slower than predicted by the formula above.

avoids distorting our analysis due to the widely varying pricing policies of semiconductor vendors. Using chip area in λ^2 as an estimate of cost is a useful first approximation.

4.2   Choose the minimum granularity that provides adequate memory bandwidth

As processors represent a small fraction of the silicon area in a machine, the amount of memory per node determines the granularity. The best cost/performance is achieved at the minimum memory capacity that provides adequate memory bandwidth. That is, multiple memory components should not be multiplexed on the same data lines. Since bandwidth is the critical commodity, every memory data pin should be kept busy every cycle. Given such a *one deep* memory organization, the memory capacity of a processing node becomes the product of the width of the memory interface and the capacity per pin.

The width of the memory interface should be set at the minimum level that supports an achievable level of instruction-level-parallelism while maintaining high memory duty factor. The goal is not to maximize processor utilization, but rather to maximize memory bandwidth utilization. The MIT M-Machine uses a single word (64-data bits) wide memory interface. A narrower interface, would incur a latency penalty with multiple cycles required to fetch a word. Unless the majority of an application's memory operations are on very small data types, there is no advantage to building a memory interface (or a processor) that is less than a full word wide. A machine with a cost-balanced processor should have no trouble saturating a one-word-wide interface. An interface much wider than a single word suffers from low duty factor as spatial locality falls off. Increasing the interface width beyond two words increases cost linearly while providing a very small improvement in performance.

With the M-Machine's 1Mx16 SDRAMs, a word-wide memory is 8MBytes. As DRAM density increases, larger capacities will be required to achieve adequate bandwidth. With 16-bit wide parts, a word wide memory will be 32Mbytes with 64Mbit parts in '97 and 128MBytes with 256Mbit parts in '00. The cost of this bandwidth drives the machine far out of balance. The eventual solution is to integrate the processor on the same chip as the memory capturing this bandwidth on-chip where it is inexpensive. A major impediment to this integration is the divergence of logic and memory semiconductor processes. However, by the time 256Mbit parts arrive, the cost imbalance should be large enough to motivate manufacturers to overcome this barrier.

The issue of granularity is largely independent of processor organization. The area required by a word-wide memory today ($6.7G\lambda^2$) is sufficiently large that a fully pipelined 64-bit processor with floating point can be realized in a small fraction (5%) of the memory area. The real question is how many parallel pipelined floating-point units should be provided. The M-Machine provides four floating-point units and eight integer units bringing the area of the processor up to about 25% of the total.

Many computer users today are asking computer manufacturers for node memories much larger than the 8MB of a one-deep word-wide memory. Their motivation is to cover deficiencies in the global communication and mechanisms of the machine. Some existing parallel computers with poor network bandwidth and long message latencies (10s of μs which is 1000s of instruction times) need large node memories to perform well. If a parallel machine has sufficient network performance to be a good sequential machine (see Section 2) there is no advantage to large node memories, and considerable disadvantage due to imbalance. Similarly, approaches in which nodes are clustered are not required if the global interconnection network is adequate to meet the constraint of Section 2.

Another motivation for *fat nodes* with greater than word-wide memories is to operate on vectors in parallel. However, with adequate synchronization mechanisms, vector operations can be carried out in parallel across multiple nodes with equal efficiency and greater flexibility for scalar code and short vector lengths.

5. Mechanisms

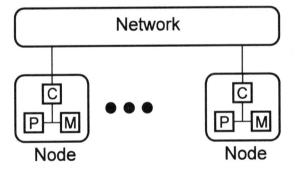

Figure 2: Block diagram of a parallel computer.

To operate with a relatively small node memory and to make effective use of global bandwidth, a parallel machine must have efficient mechanisms for communication, synchronization, and naming. All parallel computers have the basic structure shown in Figure 2. They consist of a number of nodes connected by a network. Each node contains one or more processors (P), some memory (M), and an interface to the network (C). A well-designed network should have a latency, composed of wire and switch delays, should be a few 10s of clock cycles which is comparable to the local memory access time. For example, a 1024-node J-Machine, has a maximum latency of 29clocks (about 1μs)[Da92a] , and a 256-processor Cray T3D [Cray] has a maximum network latency of 20clocks (120ns). With such networks, in the absence of contention, a processor on any node should be able to interact with another node in an amount of time equal to network latency. Thus remote memory accesses and synchronization actions should take a small multiple (2 or 3) of the local memory access time. While machines such as the J-Machine and T3D achieve these numbers, most parallel computers do not. Most parallel computers lack adequate *mechanisms* that sequence communication and synchronization and thus incur large software overheads with remote actions.

Mechanisms are the primitive operations provided by a computer's hardware and systems software. The abstractions that make up a programming system are built from these mechanisms [Da89, Da91]. For example, most sequential machines provide some mechanism for a push-down stack to support the last-in-first-out (LIFO) storage allocation required by many sequential models of computation. Most machines also provide some form of memory relocation and protection to allow several processes to coexist in memory at a single time without interference. The proper set of mechanisms can provide a significant improvement in performance over a brute-force interpretation of a computational model.

Over the past 40 years, sequential von Neumann processors have evolved a set of mechanisms appropriate for supporting most sequential models of computation. It is clear, however, from efforts to build concurrent machines by wiring together many sequential processors, that these highly-evolved sequential mechanisms are not adequate to support most parallel models of computation. These mechanisms do not support synchronization of events, communication of data, or global naming of objects. As a result, these functions, inherent to any parallel model of computation, must be implemented largely in software with prohibitive overhead.

Some parallel computers have been built with mechanisms specialized for a particular model of programming, for example dataflow, parallel logic programming, or cache-coherent shared memory. However, our studies have shown that most programming models require the same basic mechanisms for communication, synchronization, and naming. More complex model-specific mechanisms can be built from the basic mechanisms with little loss in efficiency. Specializing a machine for a particular programming model limits its flexibility and range of application without any significant gain in performance. In the remainder of this section, we will examine mechanisms for communication and synchronization. While naming mechanisms are also critical, they will not be dealt with here. The interested reader is referred to [Da91].

5.1 Efficient communication requires end-to-end hardware support.

Any communication between processing nodes involves the steps of:

Formatting: gathering the message contents together.

Addressing: selecting the physical destination for the message.

Delivery: transporting the message to the destination.

Allocation: assigning space to hold the arriving message.

Buffering: storing the message into the allocated space.

Action: performing a sequence of operations to handle the message.

All programming models use a subset of these basic steps. A shared memory read operation, for example, uses all six steps. A read message is formatted, the address is translated, the message is delivered by the network, the message is buffered until the receiving node can process it, and finally a read is performed and reply message is sent as the action. Some models, such as synchronous message passing always send messages to preallocated storage and thus omit allocation (step 4). In some cases, e.g., a remote write, no action is required to respond to a message and step 6 can be omitted.

Most parallel computers provide general hardware support only for the delivery step of a communication. The other steps, if supported at all, are hardwired for a specific model of computation, such as cache coherent shared memory. The MIT J-Machine's message driven processor (MDP) [Da87] first provided model independent support for all six steps. The MIT M-Machine provides a refined version of these mechanisms. It uses a SEND instruction to atomically transmit the contents a block of registers into the network (formatting). A global TLB is used to provide relocation and protection of message destinations (addressing). A dedicated system receive thread on the destination processor extracts the message from the network, queues it if necessary (allocation and buffering), and dispatches any actions requested by the message (action).

Providing efficient yet flexible mechanisms for communication such as a SEND instruction and dedicated receive thread permits the M-Machine to perform arbitrary remote interactions, not just a few hardwired sequences, in time comparable to the network latency.

5.2 Synchronize on data

Synchronization enforces an ordering of events in a program. It is used, for example, to ensure that one process writes a memory location before another reads it, to provide mutual exclusion during critical sections of code, and to require all processes to arrive at a barrier before any processes leave.

Any synchronization mechanism requires a namespace that processes use to refer to events, a method for signalling that an event is enabled, and a method for forcing a processor to wait on an event. Using tags for synchronization, as with the presence bits on the HEP [Smith], uses the memory address space as the synchronization namespace. This provides a large synchronization namespace with very little cost as the memory management hardware is reused for this function. It also has the benefit that data can be written and an event signaled in a single memory operation. Since it naturally signals the presence of data, we refer to this synchronization using tags on memory words as *data synchronization* [Wills].

With synchronization tags, an event is signaled by setting the tag to a particular state. A process can wait on an event by performing a synchronizing access of the location which raises an exception if the tag is not in the expected state. A synchronizing access may optionally leave the tag in a different state. Simple producer/consumer synchronization can be performed using a single state bit. In this case, the producer executes a synchronizing write which expects the tag to be empty and leaves it full. A synchronizing read which expects the location to be full and leaves it empty is performed by the consumer. If the operations proceed in order, no exceptions are raised. An attempt to read before a write or to write twice before a single read raises a synchronization exception [Da91]. Both the J-Machine and M-Machine provide presence tags for synchronization.

The communication mechanism described above complements data synchronization by providing a means for a process on one node to signal an event on a remote node. In the simplest case, a message handler can perform a synchronizing read or write operation. However, it is often more efficient to move some computation to the node on which the data is resident. Consider for example the problem of adding a value to a remote location. This occurs, for example, when performing LU decomposition of a matrix. One could perform a remote synchronizing read that marks the location empty to gain exclusive access, perform the add, and then perform a remote synchronizing write. Sending a single message to invoke a handler that performs the read, add, and write on the remote node, however, reduces the time to perform the operation, the number of messages required, and the amount of time the location is locked.

Hardwired shared memory machines lack the ability to have a message handler signal the arrival of data or carry out a remote computation. These machines have all the datapaths required for these operations, but their controllers are hardwired a few message actions rather than providing for the generality of a handler. This deficiency of specializing the mechanisms for a model of computation costs many redundant messages during synchronization operations.

The mechanism that enforces event ordering solves only half of the synchronization problem. Efficient synchronization also requires an *agile* processor that can rapidly switch processes and handle events and messages to reduce the exception handling and context switching overhead when switching processes while waiting on an event. The M-Machine uses multithreading to achieve agility. Each M-Machine node multiplexes sixteen user *H-Threads* along with eight dedicated system H-Threads. Separate, dedicated resident threads are used to handle arriving messages, local memory system events, and pipeline exceptions making the handling of these conditions very rapid.

6. Conclusion

This paper has presented a set of guidelines for parallel computer design. System bandwidth should be tapered from the local to the global level according to cost and application demand. The grain size of the system should be chosen to maximize memory bandwidth. The division of resources within each node should be driven by cost and performance, not ratios of capacity to speed. Finally, efficient mechanisms enable nodes to work together at rates limited by their datapath delays.

Bandwidth is the critical resource in any computer system. In a parallel computer system, bandwidth must be managed to optimize the cost/performance. The locality of applications can be exploited by providing abundant inexpensive local bandwidth and less of the expensive global bandwidth. Global bandwidth will determine application performance. However, this expensive resource can be kept busy by oversupplying the inexpensive resource.

The cost of a node should be divided between the processor and memory to equalize the incremental gain per unit cost, $\partial P/\partial c_p = \partial P/\partial c_m$. Because the cost of a modern computer is dominated by memory, cost balance can be approximated by allocating a fraction of the node's cost (5-25%) to the processor. This is more than enough area to build a processor that can saturate the available memory bandwidth.

To optimize memory bandwidth, the grain-size of a node should be chosen to be that required to provide a one-deep memory of one or two words wide. Deeper memories squander the pin bandwidth of the DRAMs by multiplexing them together. Wider memories suffer from reduced spatial locality and poor performance on non-unit-stride accesses. Narrower memories increase latency and reduce sequential performance. As DRAM technology scales, the capacity of memories will grow larger than their bandwidth can support. Bandwidth-limited node memories will be forced to use more capacity than required to achieve adequate bandwidth. Eventually the high cost of using component pin bandwidth to connect a processor to its local memory will drive manufacturers to put the processor on the memory chip despite divergent logic and memory technologies.

To realize the performance gains of parallelism overheads must be reduced by using efficient yet flexible communication and synchronization mechanisms. A processor with end-to-end hardware support for communication can interact with a remote node in time comparable to the network latency. Making this support programmable, by dispatching a message handler at the remote node, for example, allows it to be used for arbitrary remote actions. Specializing communication for one model of computation may result in excess use of network bandwidth. To synchronize with operations on remote nodes, processors must support synchronizing operations on memory and must be agile, able to switch tasks quickly when a synchronizing operation fails.

There are several important computer design issues that have not been covered in this paper. For example, low network latency is important to realizing the goal of good sequential performance. However, for most machines, the latency of the network is dominated by the latency of the mechanisms used to interface with the network. Providing high-performance symmetric input/output (I/O) is important to system performance. However, the bandwidth demands for I/O are low compared to the global communication bandwidth of a system and the I/O can piggyback on the interconnection network provided for global communication.

The rapid, exponential increase in circuit density promises to make parallel computers pervasive. As chip densities increase beyond that required to build a pipelined superscalar processor, designers must use explicit parallelism to convert density to performance. Such machines will be memory and communication bandwidth limited. Arithmetic performance is inexpensive, inter-chip bandwidth and especially global bandwidth are the critical resources. The memory bandwidth bottleneck will eventually force manufacturers to integrate processors on the memory chip despite divergent process technologies. The resulting processor-DRAM chip will be the building block for computers ranging from desktop PCs to the most powerful supercomputers. To build these machines the designers must effectively manage the bandwidth hierarchy, balance their nodes by cost, and use efficient mechanisms for communication and synchronization.

References

[Cray]   Cray Research, *Cray T3D Technical Overview*, 1993.

[Da86]   Dally, William J. "Directions in Concurrent Computing, *Proceedings of the International Conference on Computer Design*, 1986, pp. 102-106.

[Da87]   Dally, William J., et. al., "Architecture of a Message-Driven Processor," *Proceedings of the 14th International Symposium on Computer Architecture, 1987*, pp. 189-205.

[Da89]   Dally, William J. and Wills, D. Scott, "Universal Mechanisms for Concurrency," *Proceedings of Parallel Architectures and Languages Europe, 1989*, Springer Verlag, pp. 19-33.

[Da91]   Dally, William J.,Wills, D. Scott, and Lethin, Richard, "Mechanisms for Parallel Computing", *Proceedings of the NATO Advanced Study Institute on Parallel Computing on Distributed Memory Multiprocessors*, 1991, Springer-Verlag.

[Da92a]   Dally, William et. al, "The Message-Driven Processor: A Multicomputer Processing Node with Efficient Mechanisms", *IEEE Micro*, April 1992. Vol. 12, No. 2, pp. 23-39.

[Da92b]   Dally, "A Universal Parallel Computer Architecture", *New Generation Computing*, June 1993.

[DLD93]   Dennison, Larry R., Lee, Whay S., and Dally, William J., "High-Performance Bidirectional Signalling in VLSI Systems", *Proceedings of the 1993 Symposium on Research on Integrated Systems*, March 1993, MIT Press, pp. 300-319.

[HP90]   Hennessy, John L. and Patterson, David A., *Computer Architecture: A Quantitative Approach*, Morgan Kaufmann, 1990.

[HJ91]   Hennessy, John L. and Jouppi, Norman P., "Computer Technology and Architecture: An Evolving Interaction, *Computer*, September 1991, pp. 18-29.

[KD92]   Keckler, Stephen W. and Dally, William J., "Processor Coupling: Integrating Compile Time and Runtime Scheduling for Parallelism", *Proceedings of the 19th International Symposium on Computer Architecture*, 1992, pp. 202-213.

[MC78]   Mead and Conway, *Introduction to VLSI Systems,* Addison Wesley, 1978.

[Smith]   Smith, Burton J., "Architecture and Applications of the HEP Multiprocessor Computer System", *SPIE Vol. 298 Real-Time Signal Processing IV,* 1981, pp. 241-248.

[YDA94]   Yeung, Donald, Dally, William J., and Agarwal Anant, "How to Chose the Grain Size of a Parallel Computer," Submitted for publication.

[Wills]   Wills, D. Scott, *Pi: A Parallel Architecture Interface for Multi-Model Execution*, Sc.D. Thesis, Massachusetts Institute of Technology, 1990.

Chapter 9
RWC Massively Parallel Computer Project
—RWC Architecture—

Shuichi Sakai*

Abstract

This paper presents the basic architecture of the massively parallel computer which is being developed by Real World Computing (RWC) Program in Japan. The purposes of this research and development are to efficiently support flexible and integrated information processing which are research targets in RWC, and to pursue a general purpose stand-alone massively parallel system efficiently supporting multiple programming paradigms. For this purpose, a rational system is now under development with a strong collaboration among hardware people, software people and application people.

The architectural features of this system are: (1) continuation driven execution model where massively parallel execution is naturally expressed both for hardware and software. (2) Reduced Interprocessor–Communication Architecture (RICA) where communication, scheduling and instruction execution are tightly integrated. (3) support for a massively parallel operating system. (4) a cube connected circular banyan interconnection network, and (5) an independent I/O network.

This paper describes the approaches of the RWC massively parallel system project, briefly examines the above features, and shows the near future plan for machine development.

1   Introduction

The Real World Computing Program (RWC Program) is a MITI ten year international project whose budget will be about 60 billion yen (about US$550,000,000) [1]. One of its research topics is massively parallel computation [4]. The purposes for the research and development of the RWC massively parallel computer project are as follows.

1. To efficiently support flexible and integrated computation which are research targets in the RWC Project.

---

*Massively Parallel Architecture Laboratory, Real World Computing Partnership, Tsukuba Mitsui Building 16F, 1-6-1 Takezono, Tsukuba, Ibaraki 305, Japan. Phone: +81-298-53-1650. Fax: +81-298-53-1652 EMAIL: sakai@trc.rwcp.or.jp

Examples of the "flexible and integrated computation" are (1) information processing where patterns and symbols are integrated, (2) neural computation and (3) flexible autonomous control of robots.

2. To pursue a general purpose massively parallel system efficiently supporting multiple programming paradigms.

   The application fields include numerical applications and parallel symbolic processing in addition to the flexible and integrated computation.

3. To realize a stand-alone system which has a mature operating system.

   The machine should take a central role in a computational infrastructure in RWC. It should provide high-quality services as well as computation speed. It is necessary to provide data protection and excellent response time under a multiple-user multiple-process environment.

4. To support time-dependent execution.

   One of the main goals of RWC is to give appropriate answers to real world problems in a meaningful time. The typical case is a robot control where visual and phonetic information must be processed in a real time.

Two research fields, architecture and software, are strongly coupled and are collaborating to approach these goals. The overall research topics are as follows.

1. massively parallel execution model and massively parallel architecture

2. operating systems for massively parallel systems

3. languages for massively parallel systems

4. environments for system development and programming

5. system evaluation.

This paper will mainly present the approaches from the architecture side [2]. Section 2 describes the execution model for the RWC massively parallel system. Section 3 presents the processor architecture where computation and communication are tightly fused for exploiting fine grain parallelism. Section 4 shows how the architecture supports massively parallel operating systems. Section 5 introduces the interconnection network. Section 6 briefly describes the RWC massively parallel software, and shows the plan for machine development.

Note that this paper concentrates on the research at RWC Tsukuba Research Center (TRC), a central laboratory of RWC. There are other distributed laboratories in RWC, i.e., NEC Lab., SANYO Lab., Toshiba Lab., Mitsubishi Lab., Mitsubishi Research Institute's Lab. and GMD Lab.

2   Continuation-Driven Execution Model

2.1   Requirements for the Execution Model

The execution model defines how activities are invoked, how they are executed and how they are terminated. It should provide both the abstract architecture for a hardware design that is feasible and efficient, and the basis for natural and facile mapping from programs to processor architecture.

To satisfy these requirements, we propose a *Continuation-Driven Model* as an execution model. The exact definition and detailed examination of this model were described in another paper [3], so this paper will briefly present this model and show its features.

2.2   Continuation-Driven Execution Model

The Continuation-Driven Execution Model is an advanced multithreaded execution model. Figure 1 illustrates the operations in the model.

In this model, a series of instructions which are continuously executed in each PE is called a *thread*. Each thread is invoked by an *activator* which is an abstraction of a message. It involves a *continuation* and a series of data. A continuation is a triplet of (pe, ip, dp) where pe is a destination processing element (PE) address, ip is an instruction pointer and dp is a data pointer. The latter two pointers are used for identifying the starting point of a thread.

The abstract process of this model has an *Activator Queue* and a *Thread Executor*. The Activator Queue holds activators waiting for firing. It does not need to be a FIFO queue, but can be a prioritized queue. The Thread Executor executes instructions in a certain thread, creates a new activator, and terminates the current thread.

The following briefly describes the execution rules of this model.

1. Thread invocation.

   Each thread is invoked by picking up the highest priority activator and passing ip and dp to an instruction address register (ia) and a data address register (da) respectively.

2. Instruction execution in each thread.

   Instruction execution is the same as that of the normal von Neumann processor, e.g. superscalar RISC processor.

3. Thread termination.

   A thread is terminated by a *break instruction* or a *break flag* which is a part of an instruction word.

4. Forks.

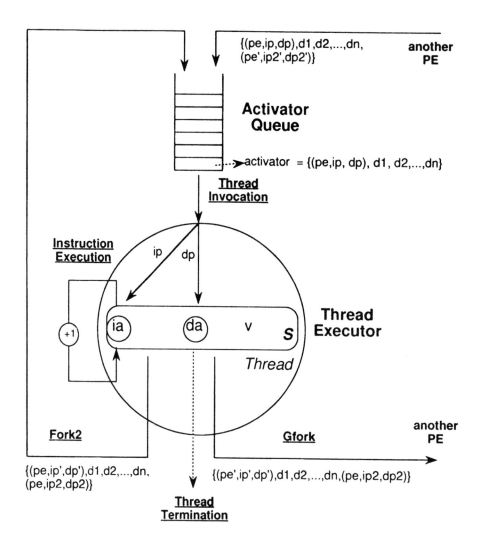

FIG. 1. *Continuation Driven Execution Model.*

A fork is implemented by creating a new activator, sending it to its destination and invoking a new thread. The activator can contain a return continuation as its data.

5. Join.

A join needs indivisible instructions for synchronization. The model typically realizes this by updating a flag and branching if successful.

6. Remote memory read and write.

A remote memory word is read and written by sending an activator which includes the memory address and return continuation. The remote PE reads (or writes) data and returns it according to the return continuation (or does not return).

7. Procedure call and return.

A procedure call is realized by a fork with a reservation of a new frame. If a value return is necessary, then the activator for the fork contains the return continuation. According to it, the return is realized by generating an activator and sending it.

This model naturally integrates the communication, scheduling, synchronization and computation.

3   Reduced Interprocessor-Communication Architecture

Based on the Continuation-Driven Execution Model, we propose the processor architecture called *RICA, Reduced Interprocessor Communication Architecture*. Figure 2 illustrates the organization of RICA.

In RICA, activators are realized in two ways: messages and local continuations. If the activator should be transferred to another PE, it is packed into a message by the message generation pipeline and automatically sent into the interconnection network. If it is transferred inside the PE, the pair of the destination instruction address and the data address is stored in the Activator Queue.

The Activator Queue is realized by a hardware priority queue. It receives messages as well as local continuations. It then supplies the activator to the Thread Executor. Note that there is no 'start' instruction for thread invocation; hardware automatically does this.

Thread invocation means passing the activator from the Activator Queue to the Thread Executor. To pass an (ip, dp) pair requires only a single cycle which is pipelined to the last instruction execution of the previous thread. As soon as the pair is set to the (ia, da), the thread instructions are fetched and decoded. They will be executed as soon as the data is set to the register under scoreboarding mechanisms. It is not necessary to wait for all data input; each data input used by the instruction enables an execution.

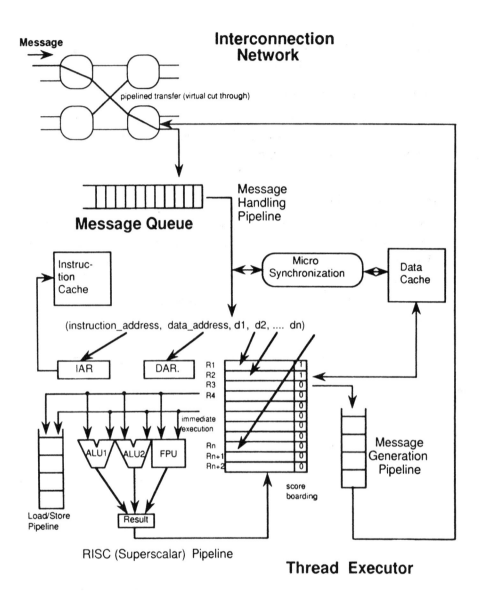

FIG. 2. *Reduced Interprocessor Communication Architecture.*

Join operations are supported by the micro-synchronization mechanisms in RICA [5]. This means a sequence of (1) test and set of the flag and (2) branch by the flag value. RICA has special hardware for supporting micro-synchronizations. This will considerably reduce the time for a Join.

Each instruction is executed in a super-scalar mechanism in a RICA Thread Executor. Each thread is terminated if it encounters *Break* instruction. Threads are quickly switched by over-lapping register load/store and thread execution. RICA provides multiple register set for this purpose.

Messages are generated by a special pipeline (operating asynchronously with other pipelines.). There is a special instruction *make_message* for it.

Briefly, the features of RICA are as follows.

1. fast and simplified message handling and message generation;

2. hard-wired queuing and scheduling mechanisms;

3. hard-wired micro-synchronization;

4. fusing communication, scheduling and computation;

5. simplifying the whole structure.

4   Support for Massively Parallel Operating System

A massively parallel operating system is necessary for an efficient and safe stand-alone computer. In RWC massively parallel project, we propose and will implement the following.

• global virtual memory and protection mechanisms

• four-level priority control

• flexible and efficient time and space sharing

• support for time-dependent processing

Among those, global virtual memory [6] will be discussed here.

We propose global virtual addressing, where PE addresses are virtualized as are local memory addresses. Ideally, the most general mapping, i.e. any gva to any (PPE, lpa) pair should be performed where gva is a global virtual address, PPE is a physical PE number and lpa is a local physical address. However, this requires an extremely huge translation table, which would be an over-specification.

RWC is now examining an indirection method called relative PE addressing. In this addressing method, gva is represented as a pair (RPE, lva) where RPE is a relative PE number and lva is a local virtual address. Each PE has a global translation look-aside buffer in the message generation circuit that translates RPE to PPE. The (PPE, lva) pair is transferred in a message header, and the destination PE translates lva to lpa as a usual memory controller does. Figure 3 illustrates the RPE translation method in comparison with other two methods.

This method reduces the size of each translation table and simplifies the translation. We are also considering an extension of the relative PE addressing where some bits of the field *lva* are used for determining *PPE*.

We are also examining the paging system for massively parallel circumstances.

5   Cube-Connected Circular Banyan Interconnection Network

An interconnection network is a performance decisive factor in a massively parallel computer. We have proposed a new interconnection network for RWC massively parallel computers. This network is called Cube-Connected Circular Banyan (CCCB) [7].

Figure 4 illustrates the CCCB. The network can be seen as a three-dimensional network. From one dimension, it can be seen as a circular banyan network. From another dimension, it can be seen as a binary cube.

The features of this network are as follows.

1. low hardware cost: $O(N)$ where N is the number of processing nodes, and the degree of each node=3;

2. high bandwidth, small delay (diameter $O(\log N)$);

3. simple self routing;

4. store-and-forward deadlock prevention by spiral buffers;

5. easy and efficient space division;

6. time division supported by draining mechanisms.

6   RWC Software and Plan for System Development

6.1   Overview of RWC Software

Figure 5 illustrates the RWC software [4]. The main software being developed in TRC are a kernel *SCore*, a description language *MPC++*, and a base language *OCore*.

SCore uses the micro-kernel technologies and efficiently realizes the minimum set of kernel functions. It exploits the architectural features of the RWC massively parallel computer and it can treat time-dependent problems as well as time sharing and space sharing.

MPC++ is an object oriented language which is an extension of C++ for distributed memory parallel computers. It is upward compatible with C

(a) Direct Complete Translation

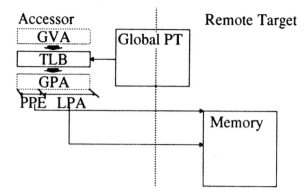

(b) Indirect Complete Translation

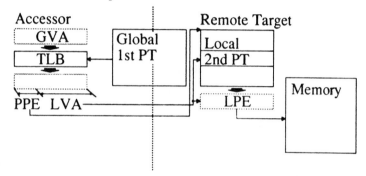

(c) RPE Translation

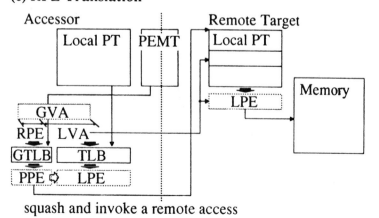

FIG. 3. *RPE Translation Method.*

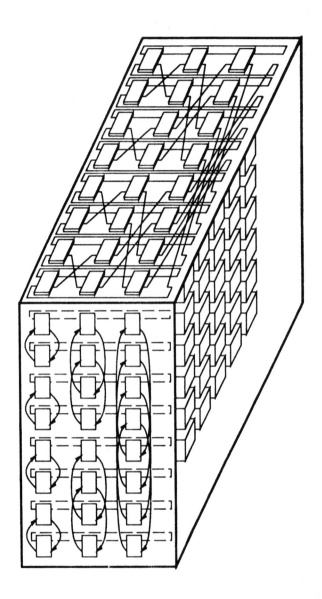

FIG. 4. *Cube Connected Circular Banyan Network.*

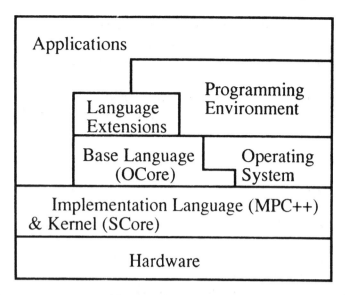

FIG. 5. *RWC Software.*

and C++ and is used by system developers and super-power users. MPC++ treats data parallelism as well as control parallelism.

OCore is a higher level object-oriented language. The features of the OCore are 1) compactness, 2) meta-level description, 3) description of time dependence and 4) massively parallel garbage collectors.

6.2   Plan for System Development

TRC is now developing the massively parallel prototype called *RWC-1*. RWC-1 will have 1,024 PEs and will be assembled in March 1996. RWC-1 is an experimental machine for proving the concepts, mechanical features and efficiency of the model. Absolute peak performance is not the purpose of this system.

RWC-1 contains original processor chips, original interconnection switches and original maintenance hardware. In the first step, we have been developing the first testbed since 1993.

In the testbed, the processor chip is made of a CMOS standard cell and the network switch is a BiCMOS gate array. The testbed with eight processors became operational with I/O and maintenance hardware in the 3rd quarter of 1994.

Until the hardware is operational, software will be developed on RWC-1 simulators. We are now developing two kinds of software simulators: instruction set level and register transfer level. The first version of the instruction set level simulator was completed in March 1994.

MPC++ was specified and the part of its first compiler, which treats control parallelism, was completed. Object code output by the MPC++

compiler is now executed on the instruction set level simulator. In addition, the basic part of the OCore was completed. The MPC++ and OCore systems will be developed on commercial parallel computers as well as RWC-1.

We also are now collecting massively parallel application programs which will be executed on RWC-1. They will be from the field of 1) RWC research for new functionality, 2) large scale simulations, 3) numerical analyses, and 4) symbolic computation.

7   Conclusion

This paper presents the basic architecture of the RWC massively parallel computer.

The architectural features of this system are: (1) continuation-driven execution model where massively parallel execution is naturally expressed both for hardware and basic software, (2) Reduced Interprocessor-Communication Architecture (RICA) where communication, scheduling and instruction execution are tightly integrated, (3) support for a massively parallel operating system, (4) a cube-connected circular banyan interconnection network, and (5) an independent I/O network.

This paper has briefly examined the above features, introduces the RWC software and shows the near future plan for the machine development.

References

[1] The Master Plan for the Real-World Computing Program, MITI Japan, pp. 30–37 (1992).

[2] Shuichi Sakai, Kazuaki Okamoto, Hiroshi Matsuoka, Hideo Hirono, Yuetsu Kodama, Mitsuhisa Sato and Takashi Yokota, Basic Features of a Massively Parallel Computer RWC-1, Proc. JSPP'93, pp. 87–94 (1993) *in Japanese*.

[3] Shuichi Sakai, Kazuaki Okamoto, Yuetsu Kodama and Mitsuhisa Sato, Reduced Interprocessor-Communication Architecture for Supporting Programming Models, Proceedings of Conference on Massively Parallel Programming Models, pp. 134–143 (1993).

[4] Shuichi Sakai and Yutaka Ishikawa, Research and Development of RWC Massively Parallel Computing Systems, Information Processing of IPSJ, Vol. 34, No. 2, pp. 1440–1444 (1993) *in Japanese*.

[5] Kazuaki Okamoto, Hiroshi Matsuoka, Hideo Hirono, Takashi Yokota, Atsushi Hori, Yuetsu Kodama, Mitsuhisa Sato and Shuichi Sakai, Synchronization Mechanisms on the Massively Parallel Computer RWC-1, Research Reports on Computer Architecture of ISPJ, 101-2 (1993), *in Japanese*.

[6] Hiroshi Matsuoka, Kazuaki Okamoto, Hideo Hirono, Takashi Yokota, Atsushi Hori, Yuetsu Kodama, Mitsuhisa Sato and Shuichi Sakai, Memory System for the Massively Parallel Computer RWC-1, Research Reports on Computer Architecture of ISPJ, 101-3 (1993), *in Japanese*.

[7] Takashi Yokota, Hiroshi Matsuoka, Kazuaki Okamoto, Hideo Hirono, Atsushi Hori, Yuetsu Kodama, Mitsuhisa Sato and Shuichi Sakai, Interconnection

Networks for the Massively Parallel Computer RWC-1, Research Reports on Computer Architecture of ISPJ, 101-4 (1993), *in Japanese*.

Index

active-dependent models, 45
afferent inputs, Monte Carlo simulation of self organization, 101
afferent projections, overall topography, 109
asynchronous parallel genetic algorithm, 142, 148
auditory system, 4
  phase-locked signals, 9
avoidance, jamming response, 3

balance a design for a parallel computer, 171
bandwidth taper, 168
bandwidth, communication, for parallel computers, 168
bapta, 61
barn owl, 4
  detection of interaural phase differences, 12
bats, echolocating, 14
blocking effect, 135
breeding digital organisms, 87
buffering mechanisms, 48
bursting, 54

calcium, 46
Calliphora vicina, 26
Cambrian explosion, 79
  digital, 82
cell culture, 58
center-type patches (CTPs), 94
  and ocular dominance columns, 104
channel insertion, 45
  modulation, 45

removal, 45
synthesis, 45
chip density, trends in, 166
chip speed, trends in, 166
classification errors, 146
CNS, time-coding in, 1
coincidence detectors, 13
columns, ocular dominance (ODC's), 94
communication bandwidth for parallel computers, 167
  hardware support for, 176
  synchronization and naming, mechanisms, 174
community diversity, 73
complex systems, 70
computation, life as a metaphor, 80
  neuroidal model of, 128
computer simulation of self-organization of afferent inputs, 100
conditioned inhibition, 135
conditioning schedule, 137
conditioning, Pavlovian, 130
conductance-based neuron models, 46
continuation driven execution model, 183, 186
contrast, 36
correlation function, presynaptic, 98
correlator model, 21
crossover, 147
CTPs (center-type patches), 94
cube connected circular banyan interconnection network, 183, 190

cytochrome c, 143

data synchronization, 177
description length, for rule complexity, 151
   of likelihood, 160
   of probabilities, 161
   of stochastic motif, 162
design issues, parallel machine, 164
detection, of interaural phase differences in the barn owl, 12
   of phase differences in electric fish, 11
   of temporal information, 2
digital "neural networks" 80
digital biodiversity reserve, 87
digital biologists, 87
digital Cambrian explosion, 82
digital organism, 77
distribution of conductances, 55
divergence, 142

echolocating bats, 14
ecological communities, 78
effects of visual experience, 111
Eigenmannia, electric fish, 2
electric fish, 2
   detection of phase differences, 11
   Eigenmannia, 2
electrosensory information, parallel processing, 5
electrosensory system, 2, 4
encoding of temporal information, 4
entropy, evolution and, 75
equilibrium potentials, 51
equivalent noise power, 33

evolution, 69
   and entropy, 75
   applications of, 85
evolutionary paths to parallelism, 165
evolutionary races, 73
external disinhibition, 137
external inhibition, 137
extinction, 134

feedback, 45
firing frequency, 50
fish, electric, Eigenmannia, 2
fitness value, calculation of, 151

Gabor function fitted to RF profiles of simple cells, 115
gain control, 56
generalization, 133
genetic algorithms, 145, 147
   asynchronous parallel, 142
   for motif extraction, 142
   parallel, 157
genetic sequences, motif extraction, 141
global virtual addressing, 189
gradient model, 26
gradient scheme, 25
granularity and balance for a parallel computer, 171
granularity, memory bandwidth, 173

H1 neuron, 28
hardware support for communication, 176
hardwired shared memory machines, communications problems of, 178
heme c binding, 143
HEP, 177

Hidden Markov Model (HMM), 142
hippocampal CA 1 pyramidal neuron, 55
horizontal collaterals, involvement of long-range, 113
Horn clauses, stochastic motif representation, 144
hyper-parasites, 74
hyperacuity for time coding, 6

inductive learning algorithms, 133
interaction function, synaptic, 98
interaural phase differences in the barn own, detection, 12
  to localize sound, 6
interconnection network, 190
intrinsic properties, 53
ion channels, 44

J-Machine, MIT, 176
jamming avoidance response, 3

Klein bottle as a representation for RF's, 115

lateral inhibition, 114
learning, 43
learning rules, Hebbian, 94
legacy, software, 165
life as a metaphor for computation, 80
light intensity, 35
likelihood, description length, 160
localize sound interaural to, phase differences, 6
long-range horizontal collaterals, involvement of, 113
long-term potentiation, 43
LP neuron, 51

M-Machine bandwidth and bandwidth cost, 168
M-Machine, MIT, 168
managing evolution, 84
massively parallel machines, 84
  operating system, 183, 189
mathematical framework for the self-organization of afferent inputs, 96
maximal conductance, 47
maximum likelihood method, MDL principle, 155
MDL learning, 145
MDL principle, 142
  and the maximum likelihood methods, 155
mechanisms for communication, synchronization and naming, 174
membrane currents, 46
memory, 43
memory bandwidth and granularity, 173
micro-kernel, 190
MIMD, 79
MIT J-Machine, 176
MIT M-Machine, 168
modulation, 44
monocular stimulation, optimal orientations, 107
Monte Carlo simulation of self-organization of afferent inputs, 100
Morris-Lecar (1981) model, 49
motif extraction, from genetic sequences, 141
  extraction, genetic algorithm, 142
  stochastic approach for, 142
  system, 148

motif representation, 149
  by Horn clauses, stochastic, 144
movement computation, 21
movement illusion, 27
movement sensitive cell, 23
MPC++, 190
multi-celluarity, 79
multi-cellular digital organisms, 81
multi-compartment neuron model, 55
multithreaded execution, 185
mutation, 73, 147

naming mechanisms for communication, synchronization, 174
natural selection, 69
network Tierra, 83
neural network models, 127
neurite outgrowth, 63
neuroidal model, 128
neuroids, 127
neuronal electrical characteristics, 44
neuronal responses to oriented bar stimuli, 104
nonlinear interactions, 33

OCore, 190
ocular dominance columns, (ODCs), 94
  and center-type patches, 104
one-point crossover, 150
one-point mutation, 150
operating system, massively parallel, 189
OPMs (orientation preference maps), 94
optimal orientations for monocular stimulation, 111

optimal performance, 22
optimal processing, 39
optimal velocity estimator, 25
organisms, multi-cellular digital, 81
orientation preference maps (OPMs), 94, 113
oriented bar stimuli, neuronal responses, 104
oriented cells, tuning curves, 111
overall topography of afferent projections, 109
overexpectation effect, 135
overfitting problems, 142, 145

parallel architectures, 79
parallel computers, granularity and balance, 171
  communication bandwith for, 168
parallel genetic algorithm, asynchronous, 142
parallel machine design issues, 164
parallel processes, 79
parallel processing of electrosensory information, 5
parallelism, evolutionary paths, 165
parasites, 73
Pavlovian conditioning, 130
phase differences in the barn owl, detection of, 12
  detection of in electric fish, 11
  interaural, to localize sound, 6
phase-locked signals in auditory system, 9
photon shot noise, 22
photoreceptor signals, 39
plasticity, 43
Potts spin variables, winner-take-all mechanisms, 96

presence tags for synchronization, 177
presynaptic correlation function, 98
probabilities, description length of, 161
protein function, 144
protein identification resources database, 152
punctuated gradualism, 75
punctuated equilibrium, 75

random access tasks, 128
Real World Computing (RWC) Program, 183
receptive field profiles, 99
receptive fields, two-dimensional structure, 105
Reduced Interprocessor Communication Architecture (RICA), 183, 187
Reichardt correlator, 25, 26
reliability, 21
representation of stochastic motifs by Horn clauses, 144
Rescorla-Wagner model, 131
response dynamics, 28
response, jamming avoidance, 3
RF profiles of simple cells, Gabor function fitted to, 115
RFs, Klein bottle as a representation of, 115
rhythmic activity, 56
RICA, Reduced Interprocessor Communication Architecture, 183, 187
rule complexity, description length, 151
RWC-1, 193

sampling errors, 145
selection, 147
selective learning, requirement of, 112
self-assembly, 50
self-generating, 70
self-organization of afferent inputs, computer simulation, 100
    mathematical framework, 96
    Monte Carlo simulation, 101
self-replicating program, 73
self-replication, 70
sensory preconditioning, 133
shared memory machines, hardwired, communications problems of, 178
sigmoidal functions, 48
signal-to-noise, 25
SIMD, 79
software legacy, 165
spatial structure, 55
spontaneous recovery, 137
spontaneously differentiated 55
stability, 48, 51
stochastic approach for motif extraction, 142
stochastic motif, 143
stochastic motif extraction by HMM, 158
    experiment results, 152
stochastic motif representation, 142
    by Horn clauses, 144
stochastic motif, description length, 162
    fitness of, 146
stomato ganglion, 53
synaptic efficacy, 63
synaptic interaction function, 98
synchronization, 177

  mechanisms for communication
    and naming, 174
  presence tags for, 177

temporal information, detection of,
    2
  encoding, 4
threshold element, classical, defi-
    nition, 127
Tierra, 72, 83
Tierra, network, 83
time coding, hyperacuity, 6
time differences, detecting, 9
time-coding in the CNS, 1
topological analysis of visual in-
    formation representation,
    115
tuning curves for oriented cells, 111
two-cell network, 54
two-dimensional structure of recep-
    tive fields, 105

virtual computer, 83
visual experience, effects of, 111
visual information, topological anal-
    ysis, 115
Volterra series, 21

winner-take-all mechanism and Potts
    spin variables, 96